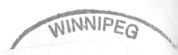

100 Questions & About Bipolar (Manic-Depressive) Disorder

Ava T. Albrecht, MD
New York University
School of Medicine

Charles Herrick, MD
New York Medical College

JONES AND BARTLETT PUBLISHERS
Sudbury, Massachusetts

BOSTON   TORONTO   LONDON   SINGAPORE

World Headquarters
Jones and Bartlett Publishers
40 Tall Pine Drive
Sudbury, MA 01776
978-443-5000
info@jbpub.com
www.jbpub.com

Jones and Bartlett Publishers
Canada
6339 Ormindale Way
Mississauga, Ontario L5V 1J2
CANADA

Jones and Bartlett Publishers
International
Barb House, Barb Mews
London W6 7PA
UK

Jones and Bartlett's books and products are available through most bookstores and online booksellers. To contact Jones and Bartlett Publishers directly, call 800-832-0034, fax 978-443-8000, or visit our website www.jbpub.com.

Substantial discounts on bulk quantities of Jones and Bartlett's publications are available to corporations, professional associations, and other qualified organizations. For details and specific discount information, contact the special sales department at Jones and Bartlett via the above contact information or send an email to specialsales@jbpub.com.

The authors, editor, and publisher have made every effort to provide accurate information. However, they are not responsible for errors, omissions, or for any outcomes related to the use of the contents of this book and take no responsibility for the use of the products described. Treatments and side effects described in this book may not be applicable to all patients; likewise, some patients may require a dose or experience a side effect that is not described herein. The reader should confer with his or her own physician regarding specific treatments and side effects. Drugs and medical devices are discussed that may have limited availability controlled by the Food and Drug Administration (FDA) for use only in a research study or clinical trial. The drug information presented has been derived from reference sources, recently published data, and pharmaceutical research data. Research, clinical practice, and government regulations often change the accepted standard in this field. When consideration is being given to use of any drug in the clinical setting, the health care provider or reader is responsible for determining FDA status of the drug, reading the package insert, reviewing prescribing information for the most up-to-date recommendations on dose, precautions, and contraindications, and determining the appropriate usage for the product. This is especially important in the case of drugs that are new or seldom used.

Production Credits
Executive Publisher: Christopher Davis
Production Director: Amy Rose
Manufacturing Buyer: Amy Bacus
Associate Editor: Kathy Richardson
Associate Marketing Manager: Laura Kavigian
Composition: Northeast Compositors, Inc.
Cover Design: Kate Ternullo
Cover Image: © Photos.com
Cover Image: © Photodisc
Printing and Binding: Malloy, Inc.
Cover Printing: Malloy, Inc.

6048

Library of Congress Cataloging-in-Publication Data
Albrecht, Ava T.
   100 questions and answers about bipolar (manic depressive) disorder / Ava T. Albrecht and Charles Herrick.
      p. cm.
   Includes index.
   ISBN-13: 978-0-7637-3231-8
   ISBN-10: 0-7637-3231-1
   1. Manic-depressive illness—Popular works. I. Herrick, Charles. II. Title. III. Title: One hundred questions and answers about bipolar (manic depressive) disorder.
   RC516.A37 2007
   616.89'5—dc22

                                2006028729

Printed in the United States of America
10 09 08 07 06   10 9 8 7 6 5 4 3 2 1

Contents

Part I: The Basics   1

Questions 1-10 give background information about bipolar disorder with such topics as:

- How does the brain affect behavior and regulate emotional states?
- What is bipolar disorder?
- What causes bipolar disorder?

Part II: Diagnosis   29

Questions 11-24 outline the steps in determining whether you have bipolar disorder, including:

- What are the symptoms of bipolar disorder?
- How is bipolar disorder diagnosed?
- Are there different types of bipolar disorder?
- How does bipolar depression differ from major depression?

Part III: Risk/Prevention/Epidemiology   57

Questions 25-34 explore details of bipolar disorder, such as:

- What are the risk factors for development of bipolar disorder?
- Are people from different ethnic backgrounds more susceptible to bipolar disorder?
- Is there a link between epilepsy and bipolar disorder?
- I have been treated for bipolar depression in the past. Can I prevent an episode in the future?

Part IV: Treatment   77

Questions 35-66 discuss the methods for treating bipolar disorder and concerns about medications, including:

- What are the different types of treatment for bipolar disorder?
- What are the different types of talk therapies and what do they do?
- What are the different types of medication used to treat bipolar disorder? How does my doctor choose a medicine?
- Can I take other medicines while I am on an antidepressant?
- Are there long-term dangers to taking medication?

After completing our first book, entitled *100 Questions & Answers About Depression*, it was only natural to collaborate again on a book about a mood disorder that is so commonly discussed in the media of late—bipolar disorder. Although this disorder is not as common as depression, the number of bipolar disorder diagnoses appears to be rising, mainly because of new research and consideration of symptoms that do not meet the full criteria for bipolar but do have many similar symptoms that cause significant impairment. Such symptomatology may comprise other bipolar categories that are considered part of the "bipolar disorder spectrum." Of course, as occurs with any expansion or new development of existing ideas, the psychiatric community is divided in regard to what constitutes true bipolar illness. In this book we present the data and evidence at hand, although active research continues on the subject as the DSM-V committee works toward refining diagnostic criteria for the future.

Historically, the diagnosis has been through many changes. Emil Kraeplin first described bipolar disorder, also known as manic-depressive disorder, in the early twentieth century. Prior to that, the condition was characterized as cyclic psychosis. The term was prompted, in large part, by the curious phenomena that some patients with a psychotic illness recovered fully and then relapsed in a cyclic nature, while others appeared to deteriorate slowly over time. Physicians were puzzled by this difference, and Kraeplin, through careful observations, determined that it was not so much a psychotic disorder as it was a mood disorder. Despite this reclassification, American psychiatry lagged behind its European counterparts in making this fundamental distinction. It was not until the late 1970s and early 1980s that the distinction in America was complete, partly because of the reintroduction of lithium into the

American pharmacopoeia and partly because of the work of two American psychiatric researchers, Harrison Pope and Joseph Lipinsky, that distinguishing between schizophrenia and manic depression became more than just an academic curiosity. This distinction now had real treatment implications, as the treatment of schizophrenia required lifelong antipsychotic medication while manic-depressive disorder could be managed more safely and effectively with lithium alone.

When Dr. Herrick was in training in the mid to late 1980s, the emphasis in making a diagnosis was on not mistaking manic depression for schizophrenia. Since the late 1990s, however, manic-depressive disorder has been called bipolar disorder and is solidly ensconced as a mood disorder, with little to no concern that clinicians will misdiagnose it as schizophrenia. The concern nowadays is the possibility of mistaking the disorder for unipolar depression and other psychiatric conditions such as personality disorders or drug and alcohol abuse. Why did the change of emphasis occur? The answer is long and complicated. In brief we offer several reasons:

Psychiatry's understanding and characterization of bipolar disorder has changed. For example, bipolar II disorder and childhood bipolar disorder did not "exist" in the 1980s.

The explosion of psychiatric medications into the marketplace has exposed more patients to medications that had both positive and negative effects on their moods, allowing for a broadening of psychiatry's understanding of mood disorders and how they could be pharmacologically "manipulated." For example, the SSRIs, because of their relative ease of use and tolerability, have been used more widely than their counterparts, the tricyclics. The growing numbers of patients asking for and receiving these medications was followed by greater numbers of persons being unwittingly switched into manic or hypomanic episodes, thereby leading to a change of views within the profession about the nature of mood disorders. In addition, the atypical antipsychotics, also because of their relative safety and ease of use, were found to help patients with "mood swings" that did not respond to SSRIs and who were otherwise not viewed to warrant treatment with traditional mood stabilizers.

Because of larger cultural changes in a variety of areas affecting psychiatry, the importance in distinguishing between these other psychiatric disorders is more complete. These changes occurred in deinstitutionalization, commitment laws, and, most notably, de-stigmatization of certain psychiatric conditions. Having the likes of Jane Pauley and Brooke Shields talk openly about their own strug-gles with mental illness has gone far toward people accepting the idea that these are real diseases in need of medical care. Deinstitu-tionalization and commitment laws have changed the types of patients hospitalized in psychiatric settings. Commitment laws now emphasize dangerousness rather than the presence of psychi-atric symptoms. Increasing numbers of patients are being admitted primarily with impulsive aggression, whether it is directed toward themselves or others, rather than merely because they are depressed or psychotic. Many of these patients have underlying personality disorders and substance abuse disorders. This has radically changed the focus of psychiatric care from treating psychotic illness to treat-ing explosive moods and behavior. A greater degree of overlap now exists between bipolar disorder and impulsive aggression than between bipolar disorder and schizophrenia, which has become increasingly an ambulatory condition managed primarily in the community.

Each of these changes, whether it is the number of medications available, new scientific understanding, broadening of the classifi-cation of the disorder, commitment laws, or destigmatization, has led to larger numbers of patients being diagnosed with bipolar dis-order, as well as greater interest in understanding what the condi-tion is and how it is best treated. Hopefully, this book will address the myriad questions you may have about this most curious condi-tion and its dizzying array of presentations—and more dizzying numbers of medications used in treating it.

Ava T. Albrecht, MD
Charles Herrick, MD

On August 31st, 1962, Scott Weinmann was born in Lansdale, PA. His mother, married three days shy of one year, was all of 19 years old. Raised in Queens, NY, and attending the Bronx High School of Science, Scott was the typical early overachiever. A straight "A" student throughout elementary and middle school, Scott enjoyed his middle-class upbringing. Scott attended SUNY Stony Brook, where he met the woman who became his wife 4½ years later. Scott and his wife have been working on their relationship since 1987, when they began couples therapy in Los Angeles. In 1998, Scott became enraged by something his wife said and played out a scenario that his wife had seen too many times before. Prone to fits of rage, particularly at home, Scott's wife walked on eggshells as a result. Never certain if she would trigger Scott's rage, she tried to choose her words wisely, but the task was arduous. This particular day was different, as Scott became acutely aware that something was not right with him. He recalls feeling the rage overwhelm him that afternoon and describes the sensation as, "Literally unable to control the rage that was coming over me." Scott felt it physiologically and knew that he couldn't continue living that way. Psychiatric consultation revealed the diagnosis` of bipolar disorder. After he was prescribed medication, he and his wife reported a dramatic change in Scott's mood and character, claiming symptoms remain under control as long as he stays on his medication. No longer worried about his hair-trigger responses, his wife is able to communicate with him more effectively. Their relationship has grown closer, and he is much happier with the behavior he is modeling for his children—moderate, tolerant, and compassionate. Today Scott works as a subject matter expert in IT process automation at a

Fortune 20 technology firm. He and his wife have been married 21 years and have two wonderfully inquisitive daughters, 11- and 16-years-old, and a golden retriever named Kaya. They make their home on Long Island.

Leslie McCormack suffered from the effects of bipolar disorder for 15 years prior to being diagnosed in her early 30s. Over the years many people were affected by the manifestation of her illness and she would like to apologize to each of them.

"Heartfelt thanks belong to Lois for her guidance and support, and to Sharyn, for lovingly remaining by my side throughout."

PART I

The Basics

What exactly are emotions and
why do we have them?

What is the difference between
thoughts and feelings?

How does the brain affect behavior and
regulate emotional states?

More . . .

1. What exactly are emotions and why do we have them?

Emotions are difficult to describe. Many dictionaries refer to feelings or moods when defining the word *emotion*, which further begs the question of what they are. Scientists who attempt to study emotional phenomena characterize them in terms of their particular interest, and thus definitions change depending on whether the scientist is studying the biological basis, psychological basis, or social basis of emotions. This, of course, further complicates the understanding of emotions.

Historically, the mind was thought to be separate from the body and part of the soul. In fact, "*psyche*" is the Greek root for the word *soul*. With the advent of a more scientific understanding of the brain and mind, some scientists attempt to liken the mind to software and the brain to hardware. In actuality, however, it is not quite so simple. Every change in thought, feeling, perception, or action is accompanied by a simultaneous change in brain activity. Today, scientists increasingly appreciate the fact that there is no sharp demarcation between the brain and the mind.

Despite the fact that mind and brain are essentially unified, drawing a boundary between the two allows for practical differences between them to be conceptualized in everyday lives. For example, such a boundary permits distinction between acts and motives. Distinguishing acts from motives helps with negotiation through everyday social interactions. Consider how you would feel if someone stepped on your toes. With the immediate sensation of pain you might feel shock, surprise, and probably anger, and you might immediately wonder about the person's motives or state of mind. Your response is guided by your feelings. Emotions therefore serve to engage the body to act in some manner, and the manner upon which an action is taken usually carries some survival value to a given individual.

Thus, lack of emotions could be likened to the lack of physical pain sensation. You would be numb to the environment and thus have problems interacting within it appropriately. Without the ability to feel anger, joy, sorrow, fear, or love, you would be incapable of generating priorities to action. Emotions help you to prioritize—to decide when to act and when not to act. Without such abilities, choosing between arrays of decisions you confront on a daily basis would be unfeasible.

2. What is the difference between thoughts and feelings?

Emotions or feelings are often distinguished from thoughts. Emotions are typically considered the irrational or animal part of humans, while thoughts are the rational part. Strong feelings such as anger, joy, fear, and sadness result in behaviors that do not seem to always serve one's interests. Thoughts are the words in the head that give mental content to hopes, dreams, and desires. Thoughts allow you to reason and weigh options so you can assess consequences before taking actions.

Scientists now know through experiments and clinical observation that thoughts, feelings, and perceptions coexist as a unified whole and cannot be easily teased apart. Thus every thought is given a positive or negative emotional valence that allows us to prioritize our actions upon those thoughts. Evidence in support of that comes from the fields of neurology and the computer sciences. **Neurological** studies have shown that people who suffered brain damage that cut thoughts off from feelings are unable to prioritize a list of preferences and act upon them in order to achieve even the simplest of goals. Even a simple task, like choosing a restaurant, is impossible for such people because they are trapped in a never-ending cost-benefit analysis of numerous and conflicting options. Computer programmers have similarly struggled to develop simple **algorithms** that can generate decisions appropriately weighing costs and benefits without becoming buried underneath an infinite loop of ones and zeros. Emotions are therefore a necessary piece that works with thoughts in decision making and hence planning of future goals.

3. How does the brain affect behavior and regulate emotional states?

The complex interaction between various brain components and the environment regulates emotions in a feedback loop that allows for both the environment to impact brain structure and function and the brain to impact on the environment through action. More than being a two-way street, though, the brain is more like a superhighway consisting of a variety of environmental inputs (some of which are available to our consciousness but many of which are not) and our ultimate responses to those inputs. Environmental inputs available to our consciousness are those we typically associate with the five senses: sight, smell, taste, hearing, and

Neurological

referring to all matters of the nervous system that includes brain, brain stem, spinal cord, and peripheral nerves. Problems with specific, identifiable pathophysiological processes are generally considered to be neurological as opposed to psychiatric. Problems with elements of both pathophysiological and psychiatric manifestations are considered to be neuro-psychiatric.

Algorithm

a sequence of steps to follow when approaching a particular problem.

touch. The mere words conjure up a myriad of emotional memories for past experiences. A certain odor or song can suddenly take a person back to a previous relationship or situation. The connection between a current environmental cue and memories are due to actual structural changes in the brain. In fact, long-term memories are long term because of those structural changes. The brain is not a computer but a dynamic organ capable of physical change throughout one's life.

Although sensory inputs are generally obvious, a multitude of environmental inputs occur without conscious awareness. The brain is constantly monitoring our body's internal environment—the available nutrients and chemicals, blood pressure, pulse, temperature, and respiration—and adjusts itself accordingly. It is also monitoring the external environment in ways that are not immediately apparent. These unconscious inputs can affect the emotional state in ways that are not always obvious.

Interpretations of these inputs that prompt actions are also influenced by two important factors influencing the brain long before inputs are received. Built into the brain are sets of biases, some of which are determined by **genes** and the biological (uterine) environment in which development occurs, and others by past experiences. Although genes do not cause behavior, they are the foundation for a person's entire organic makeup. Genes code for proteins, and proteins are the building blocks for both the structure and function of the human organism. Genes guide **neuroanatomy,** and in turn neuroanatomy and **neurophysiology** guide actions. Past experiences, on the other hand, are carved

Gene

DNA sequence that codes for a specific protein or that regulates other genes. Genes are heritable.

Neuroanatomy

the structural makeup of the nervous system and nervous tissue.

Neurophysiology

the part of science devoted specifically to the physiology, or function and activities, of the nervous system.

Neuronal plasticity

the act of nerve growth and change as a result of learning.

Mental illness

a medical condition associated with changes in thoughts, moods, and behaviors.

Constitution

referring to a person's biopsychological make-up—that is, personality and traits.

Basal ganglia

a region of the brain consisting of three groups of nerve cells (called the caudate nucleus, putamen, and the globus pallidus) that are collectively responsible for control of movement. Abnormalities in the basal ganglia can result in involuntary movement disorders.

Limbic system

the part of the brain thought to be related to feeding, mating, and most importantly to emotion and memory of emotional events. Brain regions within this system include the hypothalamus, hippocampus, amygdala, and cingulate gyrus as well as portions of the basal ganglia.

into the brain through a process known as **neuronal plasticity**. Nerves are pruned away like tree branches through learning and experience as the brain attempts to create more efficient and faster communication pathways through those repeated experiences. The nature of genetics and developmental experiences cause people to respond to the environment in certain ways. Although bias can predispose people toward negative actions and may be one of the mechanisms behind the development of some types of **mental illness**, it is merely biology's way of simplifying behavioral strategies to create more rapid and efficient action. Without emotions you cannot prioritize; priorities to action must be linked to a preconceived template of what you consider important in decision making. This bias is based on your emotional experiences and **constitutional** nature (genes and non-genetic biological effects).

In terms of defining the specific areas of the brain, or the anatomical locations, that control emotions, the division of regions is not clear-cut. One of the oldest and easiest to understand (but not necessarily the most accurate) theories divides the brain into three regions or layers. The most primitive is the brain stem and **basal ganglia**, followed by the **limbic system**, and then the rational brain composed of the cortex. The first layer, the brain stem, is responsible for self-preservation. It is where the "**fight or flight**" response is generated in response to perceived danger. The brain stem is also where control of certain **visceral** or "vegetative" functions (sleep, appetite, libido, heart rate, blood pressure, and so on) are generated. The limbic region (from the Latin word "*limbus*" for ring, or surrounding, because it forms a kind of border around the brain stem) is better known as the reward center, where emotions or feelings like anger, fear, love, hate, joy, and sadness originate. The limbic system is also responsible for some aspects of personal identity as related to the emotional power of memory. The third cerebral region is considered the "rational brain," capable of producing symbolic language and developing intellectual tasks such as reading, writing, and performing mathematical calculations. These neuroanatomical distinctions are really not that distinct but instead function as a unified whole, such that an assumption cannot be made of any one system taking priority over the other. The notions of brain regions as "primitive versus advanced" and "inferior versus superior" have not been supported by modern science. Brain structures are not hierarchical but egalitarian. Brain function is more akin to an orchestra than a military command center, as each component is required for the entire symphony to work, and the conductor is merely a "ghost in the machine."

Fight or flight
a reaction in the body that occurs in response to an immediate threat. Adrenaline is released, which allows for rapid energy to run (flight) or to face the threat (fight).

Visceral
a bodily sensation usually referencing the gut.

4. What exactly is mental illness? What is a major mental illness?

Before **mental illness** can be defined the concept of illness needs to be understood more completely. As medicine has become increasingly driven by techno-logical advances, the concept of disease has supplanted the concept of illness. Medicine is driven by a need for objective evidence and removal of subjective experi-ence. Although subjective data can help inform our understanding of diseases, by their very nature they are inherently unreliable. In contrast, objective, experi-

Mental illness
a medical condition defined by functional symptoms with as yet no specific patho-physiology that impairs social, aca-demic, and occupa-tional function.

The Basics

mental approaches to various diseases and their treatments have led to major advances. With the cost of health care skyrocketing, making health care dollars less and less available to treat any given disease, simple economic necessity dictates that we spend money on things that yield results. With a finite number of dollars, money is therefore spent on diseases that are more likely to be defined and cured.

Humans, however, are more than just their diseases. To be human is to experience a disease in your own unique way, different from anyone else. To be human with a disease is to suffer from an illness. Having an illness is a subjective experience that may be easily dismissed as less important than the objective facts of the disease. In treating individual patients, doctors address both disease and illness; one piece of that treatment is the elimination or control of the disease. Healing, on the other hand, requires more than just the elimination of disease; it requires an understanding of the individual patient's experience with the disease in the form of his or her illness.

Mental illness can be complicated to define, as it is generally based upon the subjective experience of those suffering from it. Fortunately, the field of psychiatry has experienced technological advances, and the number of effective psychiatric therapies available to treat mental illness has exploded in the past ten years. Unfortunately, although scientific theories have continued to advance our understanding of possible underlying causes of mental illness, little to no clinically useful objective evidence remains to validate the disease concept. This is why mental illness is so devastating to individuals suffering from it, and why it remains so stigmatized by those who little understand it. Consider a patient who sees her internist for a variety of physical complaints and is told (after negative test results) that her complaints are "all in her head," while a patient visiting the psychiatrist with the same array of complaints is provided with a medical explanation of her illness and feels reassured that it is "not all in her head." Webster's dictionary defines mental illness as a "disease of the mind," illustrating the struggle to identify boundaries between disease and illness, mind and body. Such a distinction has its utility but leads to the shame and stigmatization that exists for those suffering from mental illness.

Mental illness is better thought of in the less pejorative sense of being a disease, if merely for the fact that such a label brings aid and comfort to those who suffer from it. There is certainly enough biological evidence to argue strongly for this definition even if no clinical testing existed. The *Diagnostic and Statistical Manual of Mental Disorders, Fourth Edition, Text Revised* (DSM-IV-TR) does more than list a "menu" of symptoms for each disorder—it also requires the consideration of the impact those symptoms have on one's life in terms of distress and disability. In addition, a medical illness can not be the cause of the symptoms. It is the degree of symptom impact as well as the absence of a medical cause that defines the boundaries between normal variant, mentally ill, and physically ill. Defining the differences between the normal and pathological serve to avoid the subjectivity that can occur when defining illness of thought, emotions, or behavior.

Many terms thrown about today in popular culture are used to distinguish between types of mental illnesses, most of which stem from the previous discussion regarding the stigmatization and shame that accompany the diagnosis. Such terms include, but are not limited to, behavior disorder, brain disorder, minimal brain dysfunction, nervous breakdown, neurosis, psychosis, panic disorder, depression, schizophrenia, **personality disorder**, character disorder, major mental illness, minor mental illness, and "biologically-based condition." Most of these terms have more than one meaning depending upon who defines them. These terms are routinely defined by:

- Media and popular culture
- Politics that ultimately influence an insurance company's financial responsibility to pay for the treatment
- The legal system, to aid the criminal courts' decision to find someone not guilty by reason of insanity
- The psychiatric and psychological communities

First, popular culture and media often define mental illness by the idea that one is either "crazy" or not. Such terms as *"insane," "deranged," "demented," "mentally ill," "psychotic,"* and *"schizophrenic"* are most often associated with some appalling violent or criminal act that seems to lack any understandable motive that can be discovered by either the police or the press. In this situation the term *"crazy"* substitutes for the lack of apparent motive. No matter how many times the argument is made that the mentally ill are no more violent than society at large, this never stops the press from pointing out when someone is mentally ill after being arrested for a heinous criminal act. Some of these terms, such as *schiz-*

Personality disorder

maladaptive behavior patterns that persist throughout the life span that cause functional impairments.

ophrenia, do have specific psychiatric definitions that are part of the DSM-IV. Some include legal terms such as *insanity* that only the courts can determine. The media and popular culture, however, define all in pejorative terms that carry clear moral connotations. Such definitions can lead people to avoid a psychiatrist's office for fear of being labeled as "crazy" or "mentally ill."

Second, political, legal, or economic definitions of mental illnesses are meant to protect people from arbitrary actions by virtue of their illness. Such terms include *"biologically based," "behavior disorder,"* and *"insanity."* Because of the broad reach of behavior making up the definitions of mental illness where no validated biological tests exist, the potential for abuse in our social system is rife. As a result, legal and political definitions were instituted to protect individuals and organizations from that potential abuse. To protect individuals, the term *"biologically based"* was coined in order to force insurers to pay for treatment of such DSM-IV disorders as schizophrenia, major depressive disorder, and **bipolar disorder**. Alternatively, "behavior disorders" are not considered to be "biologically based" from insurers' perspective and thus are the responsibility of the individual and not subject to third-party payment. The term *"insanity"* carries a strictly legal definition that only the courts can determine. It may be informed by the fact that an individual is suffering from a mental illness, but that is only part of the equation. One may suffer from schizophrenia but rob a grocery store for purely financial reasons. He or she is not judged insane, although psychiatrists would say that he or she has a mental illness, and the popular press might call such a person "crazy."

Bipolar disorder

a mental illness defined by episodes of mania or hypomania, classically alternating with episodes of depression. There are, however, various forms the condition can take, such as repeated episodes of mania only, or lack of alternating episodes.

Definitions that interest scientists and clinicians the most are of the third type: specific operational criteria attempting to codify mental and behavioral phenomena in a pattern that has a specific etiology (cause), diagnostic symptom list (pattern), and prognosis (result). The history of attempting to classify and understand mental illness is as long as the history of medicine itself. Distinctions between "biologically based," "psychologically based," and "socially based" are relevant only insofar as attempts are made to understand each individual, biological, psychological, and social element that goes into causing each disorder. Psychiatry is not without its own arbitrary distinctions, however. Clinicians make distinctions between "major mental illnesses" and "personality disorders," classified as Axis I and Axis II diagnoses in the DSM-IV. The two axes distinguish between major mental illnesses, or states that can wax and wane with time and treatment, and personality disorders, or traits, that are generally considered to be enduring and unresponsive to biological therapies. States change. Traits endure. This distinction is one of the "useful fictions" that inform our understanding of behavior in general and mental illness more specifically. The line between state and trait is very gray, but it has allowed psychiatry to historically focus and set limits on what can be accurately defined and treated. In the past, psychiatrists considered personality disorders as not changeable and not treatable. Science has advanced, however, showing that certain elements of personality do change with time and can be improved with treatment. Insurers and the courts, however, continue to distinguish between "biologically based" versus "behavior disorder" or mentally ill versus personality disordered.

5. What is the DSM-IV-TR?

The DSM-IV-TR (*Diagnostic and Statistical Manual of Mental Disorders, Fourth Edition, Text-Revised*) is considered the standard diagnostic manual for establishing the diagnosis of various mental disorders. In its introduction a few caveats are outlined. Mental disorder implies a distinction of disorders of the mind from those of the body, an assumption no longer considered valid. The term "mental disorder" lacks a consistent operational definition that covers all situations. Categorizing specific disorders has its limitations because there are no absolute boundaries dividing one disorder from another. The criteria listed for each disorder are guidelines only and should not be applied in either a "cookbook fashion" or in an "excessively flexible" manner. Finally, the purpose of the manual is primarily to enhance agreement among clinicians and investigators and is not to imply that any "condition meets legal or other non-medical criteria for what constitutes mental disease, mental disorder, or mental disability" (See Introduction and Cautionary Statement of DSM-IV-TR).

Keep these caveats in mind, as it is easy to get caught up in a physician's diagnosis, believing it is set in stone, which it is not. As new information is acquired in treatment the diagnosis and **treatment plan** may change. Additionally, it is not uncommon for clinicians to disagree on the diagnosis because of the previous caveats. When reading the various symptoms individually it is easy to identify with many of them and jump to the conclusion that one has the described condition. Only time and the guidance of a skilled clinician who is probing and comprehensive in his or her questioning will help establish a diagnosis that leads to an effective

The Basics

Treatment plan

the plan agreed upon by patient and clinician that will be implemented to treat a mental illness. It incorporates all modalities (therapy and medication).

treatment plan. The ability to establish a diagnosis is important in developing a treatment plan that restores one's health, and if the treatment plan fails the first order of business is to reconsider the diagnosis.

6. *How do chemicals work in the brain?*

The brain is a complex organ composed of **gray matter** and **white matter**. Gray matter consists of the cell bodies of **neurons** and other support cells, and the white matter consists of long tracts of **axons** that run between the neurons. Figure 1 illustrates a neuron.

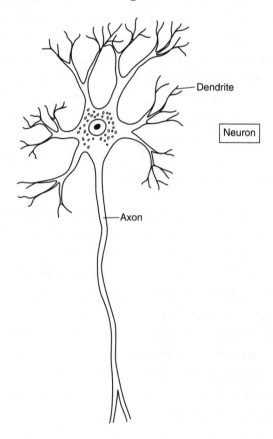

Gray matter

the part of the brain that contains the nerve cell bodies, including the cell nucleus and its metabolic machinery, as opposed to the axons, which are essentially the "transmission wires" of the nerve cell. The cerebral cortex contains gray matter.

White matter

tracts in the brain that consist of sheaths (called myelin) covering long nerve fibers.

Neuron

a nerve cell made up of a cell body with extensions called the dendrites and the axon. The dendrites carry messages from the synapse to the cell body, and the axon carries messages to the synapse to communicate with other nerve cells.

Axon

a single fiber of a nerve cell through which a message is sent via an electrical impulse to a receiving neuron. Each nerve cell has one axon.

Figure 1

Each area of the brain has a somewhat specific function. For example, the **motor cortex** controls voluntary movements of the body, and the sensory cortex processes information to the senses. Different areas of the brain communicate with other areas nearby as well as more distantly. Information travels via the axons of the neurons within the white matter areas of the brain.

The brain contains billions of neurons, which interact with each other **electrochemically**. This means that when a nerve is stimulated, a series of chemical events occur that in turn create an electrical impulse. The resulting impulse propagates down the nerve length known as the axon and causes a release of chemicals called **neurotransmitters** into a space between the stimulated nerve and the nerve it wishes to communicate with, known as the **synaptic cleft** (Figure 2). The

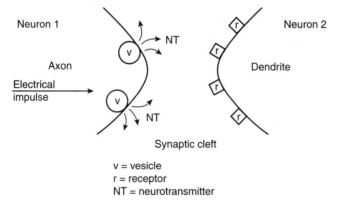

v = vesicle
r = receptor
NT = neurotransmitter

Figure 2

The Basics

Motor cortex

portion of the cerebral cortex that is directly related to voluntary movement. Also known as the motor strip, its anatomy correlates accurately with specific bodily movements, such as moving the left upper or lower extremities.

Electrochemically

the way in which signals are transmitted neurologically. Brain chemicals, or neurotransmitters, alter the electrical conductivity of nerve tissue, causing a signal to be transmitted.

Neurotransmitter

chemical in the brain that is released by nerve cells to send a message to other cells via the cell receptors.

Synaptic cleft

the junction between two neurons where neurotransmitters are released thereby continuing or changing communication.

15

Receptor

a protein on a cell upon which specific chemicals from within the body or from the environment bind, in order to cause changes in the cell that result in an electrochemical message for a certain action to be taken by that cell.

neurotransmitters interact with **receptors** on the second nerve, either stimulating them or inhibiting them. The interaction between the neurotransmitters and receptors can be likened to a key interacting with a lock where the neurotransmitter or "key" engages the receptor or "lock," causing it to "open." This "opening" is really a series of chemical changes within the second nerve that either causes that nerve to "fire" or not "fire." Thus brain activity is the result of an orchestrated series of nerves firing or not firing in binary fashion. In that sense it is much like a computer, where very complicated processes begin their lives as a series of 1s or 0s (on or off, fire or don't fire).

After the nerve fires, releasing neurotransmitters into the synaptic cleft, the neurotransmitters must be removed from the area in order to turn the signal off. There are two ways these chemicals can be removed in order to turn the signal off. The first is by destroying the chemical through the use of another chemical known as an **enzyme** with that specific purpose in mind. The second is by pumping the chemical back up into the nerve that released it by utilizing another special chemical known as a transporter or transport pump. The process of pumping chemicals back into the nerve is known as reuptake. It is important to understand these basic principles of neurophysiology because all psychoactive compounds, whether neurotransmitters, hormones, medications, or addictive drugs, involve one or more of these simple mechanisms.

Enzyme

a protein made in the body that breaks down or creates other molecules. Enzymes serve as catalysts to biochemical reactions in the body.

7. What is bipolar disorder?

Bipolar disorder, also known as manic-depressive disorder, is a medical condition of the brain that is characterized by unusual mood shifts and adversely affects a person's thoughts, feelings, and body. Also called "mood swings," these mood shifts differ from normal ups and downs in that they are associated with abnormalities in areas of sleep, appetite, energy, and libido and severely affect a person's functioning. The different mood states of bipolar disorder are treatable conditions that do not result from personal or moral weakness. The best way to characterize the mood swings of bipolar illness from normal ups and downs is to think of the term *bipolar disorder* in a global, bodily sense, where there is a reduction or activation in **physiological** activity across a variety of physical systems, including emotion and cognition. Although **stressors** can trigger an episode of depression or **mania**, a stressful life event alone does not cause the condition. Anyone is susceptible to bipolar disorder, although certain individuals are at a higher risk. Untreated bipolar disorder can evolve into a more chronic condition, with abnormal mood states becoming more and more frequent over time. As with any illness, both **morbidity** and **mortality** are associated with both the depressed and manic phases of bipolar disorder. The morbidity of either condition is the result of the **functional** impairment often experienced in areas of work, school, and relationships. The mortality of bipolar disorder is due to death by suicide or accidental death because of the functional impairments (e.g., car accident, illicit drug use, poor nutrition, neglect of health, recklessness).

The majority of people who suffer from bipolar disorder will respond to treatment, thus, it is neither warranted to suffer from depression nor wise to remain manic. Mania often feels very good to the afflicted person, while people around him or her can suffer from the manic-induced attitudes and behaviors. The

---

The Basics

Physiological

pertaining to functions and activities of the living matter, such as organs, tissues, or cells.

Stressors

environmental influences on the body and mind that can have gradual adverse effects.

Mania

a condition characterized by elevation of mood (extreme euphoria or irritability) associated with racing thoughts, decreased need for sleep, hyperactivity, and poor impulse control. One episode of mania (in the absence of an ingested substance) is needed to diagnose bipolar disorder.

Morbidity

the impact a particular disease process or illness has on one's social, academic, or occupational functioning.

Mortality

death secondary to illness or disease.

Functional

generally referring to a symptom or condition that has no clearly defined physiological or anatomical cause.

Prevalence

ratio of the frequency of cases in the population in a given time period of a particular event to the number of persons in the population at risk for the event.

Mood disorder

a type of mental illness that affects mood primarily and cognition secondarily. Mood disorders predominantly consist of depression and bipolar disorder.

lifetime **prevalence** for bipolar disorder has been deemed to be approximately 1%, although recent studies that look at the epidemiology of all bipolar spectrum conditions find figures closer to 4%. The National Institute of Mental Health (NIMH) reports that in any given one-year period, 5.7 million adults in the United States are suffering from bipolar disorder. Not only does bipolar disorder have a personal cost on individuals and their families, it has a significant cost to society. As many people who are depressed and/or manic do not seek treatment, the cost of untreated **mood disorders** to society runs into tens of billions of dollars, in part because of decreased productivity at work and overuse of primary health care services. Many individuals with bipolar II disorder or bipolar spectrum symptoms do not seek treatment but have enough functional impairment that work productivity is reduced.

Leslie's comments:

I have never experienced full-blown mania but the hypomanic state I sometimes find myself in, in contrast to depression, feels so exhilarating that it is difficult to admit that it would be better to take medication to keep this feeling in check. It is so hard to let go of the pure energy that seems to flow through my system; the feeling that anything can be accomplished. Knowing that this is a symptom of my disorder and must be kept in check is something that I grapple with whenever it occurs.

8. What causes bipolar disorder?

The causes of bipolar disorder are not easily defined. When speaking of cause, it is typical to think in terms of infections of the lungs causing pneumonia or of cigarette smoking causing lung cancer. In actuality, most medical conditions cannot be so easily defined as having clearly linked causes. In fact, it took many years of statistical analysis before scientists could demonstrate a clear causal link between cigarette smoking and lung cancer. Even today, people argue, "My grandmother smoked her entire life and died at the ripe old age of 90 from natural causes. How can cigarettes possibly cause cancer?" The reality is that cigarette smoking is only one portion, albeit a big one, of the causal puzzle that when pieced together leads to lung cancer. This is true of most diseases today. Instead, when physicians talk about cause, they are really talking about risk factors that influence the odds of developing a particular illness. For example, depression, a complex illness, is more like an illness with multiple causes that influence the odds of someone developing it. Bipolar disorder is more apt to run in families than major depressive disorder, but it also is not 100% heritable. It may occur in someone with no family history for the illness, or it may not occur in someone with extensive family history for the illness. The odds of having any mood disorder are impacted by a variety of sources inside and outside of a person. This variety constitutes what is called the **biopsychosocial** model, which is typically employed. In this model, clinicians consider biological, psychological, and social factors that may contribute to the onset of a mood disorder. This model influences most diseases of lifestyle. Take heart disease, for example. Applying the biopsychosocial model to heart disease demonstrates biological risk factors of family history, the presence of high blood pressure and high cholesterol, and atherosclerosis; psychological risk fac-

Biopsychosocial

a model used to describe the possible origins of risk factors for the development of various mental illnesses, incorporating the biological, psychological, and societal factors for a given individual.

tors of type A personality and/or an inability to handle stressful events; and social risk factors of smoking, diet, and activity level.

Biologically, bipolar disorder is associated with changes in various neurotransmitter levels and activity, commonly referred to as a **chemical imbalance** in the brain. Additionally, bipolar disorder typically runs in families, suggesting a genetic, or heritable, aspect to the illness. Psychologically, certain personality types are more prone to having less robust coping styles under stress. People who have low self-esteem and a pessimistic outlook are at higher risk for depression. Other psychological disorders, such as anxiety, psychotic, or substance abuse disorders, increase the odds of developing bipolar illness in a susceptible individual. Socially, the onset of bipolar illness is linked to stressful life events, usually entailing loss, such as of a spouse, child, job, or financial security. A mood disorder however, can also be linked to events generally considered to be uplifting rather than stressful, although from the body's reaction, they are stressful. These events can include marriage, the birth of a child, a job change or promotion, or a move to a new neighborhood or home.

Chemical imbalance

a common vernacular for what is thought to be occurring in the brain in patients suffering from mental illness.

Leslie's comments:

I remember my symptoms appearing when I was a teenager and, although I didn't link it until more recently, I am quite sure that an ongoing episode of sexual abuse during that time had a lot to do with developing the disorder. I'm also convinced that there is a genetic link because my uncle struggles with the disorder as well.

9. What chemical imbalance occurs in bipolar disorder?

Thousands of different chemicals participate in brain function and fall into different groups based on their chemical structure, mechanism of action, **psychotropic** effects, or where they come from in the body. The chemicals affecting emotional states in the brain consist of three broad types of compounds: neurotransmitters, which are chemically derived from single amino acids, the core constituents of proteins; neuropeptides, small links of amino acids that together form a protein with psychoactive effects; and hormones, chemicals made in different regions throughout the body that are released into the blood stream and also have psychoactive effects.

Neurotransmitters are chemically derived from single amino acids, the core constituents of proteins, and exist throughout the body. They are the principal actors affecting brain function, and they fall into categories based on their chemical structure. The **catecholamines** include dopamine and **norepinephrine**. The indoleamines include **serotonin**. Together these compounds make up the group **biogenic amines**. Additionally, amino acid transmitters are located in the brain in far greater quantities than neurotransmitters. Because amino acids are the building blocks of proteins used by all cells of the brain, it is difficult to demonstrate that any particular amino acid is a transmitter substance. Eight amino acids have been discovered that serve as transmitters, two of them the best understood in relation to emotion. These include glutamate, the brain's major excitatory neurotransmitter,

The Basics

Psychotropic

usually referring to pharmacological agents (medications) that, as a result of their physiological effects on the brain, lead to direct psychological effects.

Catecholamines

a class of neurotransmitters in the brain that include epinephrine, norepinephrine, and dopamine.

Norepinephrine

a neurotransmitter that is involved in the regulation of mood, arousal, and memory.

Serotonin

a neurotransmitter found in the brain and throughout the body. Serotonin is involved in mood regulation, anxiety, pain perception, appetite, sleep, sexual behavior, and impulsive behavior.

Biogenic amines

a group of compounds in the nervous system that participate in the regulation of brain activity, which includes dopamine, serotonin, and norepinephrine.

and gamma-aminobutyric acid (GABA), the brain's major inhibitory neurotransmitter.

The biogenic amines are made within small regions of the brain known as nuclei, which are concentrated areas of nerve cell bodies that act as factories of production. Axons from the nuclei in those areas of the brain act like highways that disseminate the neurotransmitters more widely throughout the brain. All three of the noted biogenic amines are involved in the regulation of mood. Dopamine, for example, is implicated in the brain's natural reward system and, therefore, is seen as pleasure generating. Norepinephrine is linked to the hormone epinephrine, also known as adrenaline. Adrenaline is associated with all risk-taking activities that cause a "rush." Serotonin was traditionally linked to activities involving sleep, appetite, and sexual function, better known in psychiatry as vegetative activities, but more recently has been implicated in control of mood and anxiety. All three biogenic amines have a large body of evidence supporting their roles in mood regulation, although ongoing research is investigating the role of various other neurotransmitters in bipolar disorder as well. Where does the evidence come from? Basically, the evidence stems from four sources: primarily from our understanding of the biological and clinical effects of various psychoactive agents on the brain; secondarily from postmortem human studies; thirdly, from experimentation with animal models; and finally, from newer imaging studies that allow mapping of neurotransmitter systems throughout the brain. Some of the evidence includes the following:

- Depletion of serotonin, norepinephrine, and dopamine (by other medications such as certain antihypertensives) can precipitate depression.

- Patients who have successfully committed suicide by violent means have evidence of reduced serotonin levels in the **central nervous system**, based on post-mortem analyses.
- **Antidepressant** medications increase the functional capacity of dopamine, serotonin, and norepinephrine to varying degrees in the brain. These medications, while effective in treating depression, can cause patients to switch into a manic state.
- Some drugs of abuse, particularly the stimulants, which increase the neurotransmitter dopamine in the brain, can trigger mania in bipolar patients and can mimic mania in non-bipolar patients.
- Some prescription medications, such as corticosteroids, used to treat various inflammatory and pulmonary diseases, can precipitate manic symptoms.
- The class of **mood stabilizers** known as the **atypical antipsychotic** medications block dopamine receptors and a subclass of serotonin receptors.
- The class of mood stabilizers known as **anticonvulsant** medications work to stabilize brain activity by increasing GABA and decreasing glutamate.
- Magnetic resonance spectroscopic imaging (MRSI), a form of magnetic resonance imaging (MRI) that allows clinicians to image not only anatomical structures but also physiologic functions. Concentrations of one particular metabolite were significantly higher in the right frontal white matter of bipolar patients compared with control subjects. In addition, two other metabolites were significantly lower in another area of the brain of bipolar patients compared with normal control subjects.

In depression, the biogenic amines are believed to be insufficient in quantity within the synaptic cleft, and

---

The Basics

Central nervous system

nerve cells and their support cells in the brain and spinal cord.

Antidepressant

a drug specifically marketed for and capable of relieving the symptoms of clinical depression. Often used to treat conditions other than depression.

Mood stabilizer

typically refers to medications for the treatment and prevention of mood swings, such as from depression to mania.

Atypical antipsychotic

a second-generation antipsychotic with a profile of targeted brain receptors that differs from the older antipsychotics, which have fewer neurological side effects and also have mood-stabilizing effects.

Anticonvulsant

a drug that controls or prevents seizures. Anticonvulsants are used in psychiatric practice to treat mania, mood instability, or other mental conditions.

thus proper communication to the receiving neuron does not occur. In mania, the biogenic amines are thought to be in too high a quantity and/or the neurons are too sensitive to their effects. Additionally, mania can be precipitated by sleep deprivation, strongly suggesting that the brain's biological clock plays a role in its development. Medications used as treatment for mania, particularly the mood stabilizers known as the anticonvulsants and lithium, stabilize the neuronal cell membranes, making them less sensitized between nerves. Additionally, many medications work by increasing the amount of GABA, the brain's major inhibitory neurotransmitter, which also makes the neurons less sensitive to stimulatory neurotransmitters. A secondary effect occurs as well. Chronic blockade of receptors with the atypical antipsychotic medications or decreased sensitivity from anticonvulsants leads to alterations in the numbers of receptors available to receive these neurotransmitters. Think of the body as continually adjusting itself in order to maintain a proper balance: any change in the system in one direction causes a change in the other direction to balance out the relationship between the two systems. This process is known in biology as **homeostasis**. **Down-regulation** or **up-regulation** of receptors is a form of homeostasis that neurons perform to compensate for any change in their availability. Such regulation requires a change in production, which is not immediate, and is perhaps one reason why mood stabilizers and antidepressants have delayed effects. A balance exists among the various chemicals involved in the regulation of signals that affect mood, and therefore bipolar disorder may be viewed partly as a chemical imbalance. Balance is restored through the use of medications that either stabilize nerve cell membranes or

Homeostasis

the maintenance of relatively stable internal physiological conditions in the body.

Down-regulation

the reduction of receptors in a region of the brain in response to increased neurotransmitter in order to maintain homeostasis.

Up-regulation

the increase of receptors in a region of the brain in response to a reduction of neurotransmitter in order to maintain homeostasis.

block neurotransmitter receptors. Keep in mind that mania is more complicated and less understood than depression and the term *chemical imbalance* represents an overly simplistic and probably erroneous though heuristically valuable notion.

Scott's comments:

The first time I became cognitively aware that I might have a psychological condition is as clear to me today as it was eight years ago when it happened. My wife said something to me in our kitchen that "pushed my buttons." The feeling that came over me was one of intense rage. I could feel the adrenaline coursing through my arteries, and I felt as though there was no way to stop this sensation. I became irate, agitated, and raised my voice. I became belligerent, and couldn't hold this outburst back. It was at that moment that I realized that I had some sort of chemical imbalance that I couldn't control using simple "mind over matter" techniques. I was cognitively aware and helpless at the same time. This event was seminal in that I sought psychiatric treatment as a direct result of this episode.

10. What is the difference between psychiatry and psychology?

Historically the sciences were considered a part of philosophy called natural philosophy because they pertained to thinkers concerned with the state of nature. Psychology was that part of natural philosophy associated with human nature. As philosophers of human nature were primarily concerned with right and wrong, psychology was considered a moral science and thus was the purview of philosophers who were contemplating the normal range of human behavior. Alternatively, abnormal behavior, more commonly known as psychopathology, was generally the purview of physicians. Those physicians were either neurologists or general practitioners whose responsibilities included the medical care of patients committed to asylums for the mentally ill. Expertise was derived primarily from exposure to those types of patients and not by any specialized training in the diagnosis and treatment of mental illness. When science separated from philosophy with the introduction of the experimental method, the field of psychology also began to adopt an equally experimental approach. Psychology retained its status in the university as an academic discipline devoted to understanding how human behavior and the mind worked.

Freud, trained as a neurologist, was the first physician to develop and describe a method of therapy whereby the patient said whatever came to mind, called **free association**. The therapist would listen critically and link up various dreams, memories, and stories the patient related to him and provide an interpretation for the patient as to the **unconscious** meanings of the patient's narrative. Through these interpretations the patient developed insight, allowing the patient to make changes in both his or her attitudes and behavior so that he or she could be relieved of pain and suffering. Freud called this method *psychoanalysis*. This was the beginning of modern psychotherapy. Freud was instrumental in expanding the treatment of mental illness in such a way as to take it out of the asylums and put it in the office. He strongly believed that although psychoanalysis required very specialized training, a medical degree was not required in order to learn and practice the technique. Thus the door was opened to psychologists becoming clinicians. Since Freud's time,

Free association

the mental process of saying out loud whatever comes to mind, suppressing the natural tendency to censor or filter thoughts. This technique is utilized in psychoanalysis and in psychodynamic psychotherapy.

Unconscious

an underlying motivation for behavior that is not available to the conscious or thoughtful mind, which has developed over the course of life experience.

universities and professional schools of psychology have expanded to train psychologists to become clinicians. Psychology students can choose a career track in either research or the practice of clinical psychology. A clinical psychologist typically has undergone four years of undergraduate education and four years of graduate education in psychology, followed by a one-year internship in a mental health care setting, treating patients under the supervision of a senior psychologist.

Psychiatrists have a radically different educational path, having grown as a specialty out of the asylum system where physicians took responsibility for the general health care of the mentally ill who were confined to asylums. Although psychology has roots in philosophy and thus a similar start in the training, psychiatrists begin studies in human anatomy and physiology as medical students. Graduating with a medical degree and the same educational background as all physicians, psychiatrists spend a year in an internship that may include psychiatry but must also include medicine or some other primary care rotation and neurology. Following internship is an additional three years as a resident physician, treating patients in a variety of settings under the supervision of a senior psychiatrist. As physicians, psychiatrists are licensed to prescribe medications, just as all physicians are. Because of their specialty, however, they develop a singular expertise in using medications to treat mental illness.

PART II

Diagnosis

What are the symptoms of bipolar disorder?

How is bipolar disorder diagnosed?

Are there different types of bipolar disorder?

More . . .

11. What are the symptoms of bipolar disorder?

When speaking of symptoms of bipolar disorder, the symptoms of concern are those of mania, specifically because bipolar disorder can be diagnosed only after a manic episode has occurred.

Signs and symptoms of mania include:

- Extremely happy, euphoric, or irritable mood
- Engagement in risk-taking behaviors
- High energy levels
- Difficulty concentrating, high distractibility
- Decreased need for sleep
- **Racing thoughts** or increased rate of speech
- Increased sex drive
- Inflated self-esteem or grandiose ideas
- Auditory or visual hallucinations
- Paranoia or delusional ideation

Racing thoughts

the subjective feeling of having thoughts in one's mind move quickly from one topic to the next, often difficult to follow and make sense of, typically associated with rapid, uninterruptible speech.

If the symptoms noted here persist for at least one week, a manic episode may be present. The greater the number of symptoms present, particularly if associated with euphoria, the more likely mania is present. Hypomania has the same symptoms, but they are judged to be less severe, need only last for four days, and are not associated with psychotic symptoms. It is also possible to have symptoms noted above in addition to such depressive symptoms as suicidal thinking, which may occur in a mixed episode, which is a combination of symptoms of mania and symptoms of major depression. Suicidal ideation warrants an immediate evaluation, as manic individuals can be extremely impulsive. Although mania is typically characterized by euphoria, severe anger and rageful mood are common as well. The decreased need for sleep is exactly a decreased *need*, which differs from **insomnia**, a condition of not being able to sleep when it is needed.

Signs and symptoms of depression occurring in a bipolar person are the same as that for major (or **unipolar**) depression and include:

- Sadness or irritability
- Loss of enjoyment of once-pleasurable activities
- Loss of energy
- Difficulty concentrating
- Insomnia or excessive sleep
- Fatigue
- Unexplained physical complaints (e.g., headache, backache, stomach upset)
- Decreased sex drive
- Change in appetite (increased or reduced)
- Feelings of hopelessness, helplessness, and/or worthlessness
- Suicidal thoughts or attempts

If the symptoms noted here persist for more than two weeks, a major depressive episode may be present, and it is more likely the greater the number of symptoms present, particularly if associated with sadness or irritability. Again, suicidal thinking warrants an immediate evaluation, especially if associated with hopelessness. Because of the multitude of physical symptoms of depression, many patients seen by a primary care health provider for certain physical complaints actually have depression. Certainly a physical evaluation to rule out any other medical conditions is warranted, but depression needs to be considered as a possible condition. If

Insomnia

the inability to fall asleep, middle-of-the-night awakening, or early morning awakening.

Unipolar

in contrast to manic-depressive illness, known as *bi*polar, or two poles of mood states, the description of major depression, or the presence of one pole of mood state.

Diagnosis

31

there is a history of mania or hypomania, a diagnosis of **bipolar depression** should be considered in the presence of such symptoms.

Bipolar depression
an episode of depression that occurs in the course of bipolar disorder.

Leslie's comments:

My symptoms began as a teenager but, unfortunately, I went undiagnosed (and therefore untreated) until my early 30s. I think because my symptoms appeared during the teen years they were easily mistaken or overlooked because they were assumed to be part of the "normal" growing pains associated with that period of one's life. I experienced severe depression for extended periods of time along with times of great energy and motivation, as if I could do(and wanted to do)anything. I would swing between these feelings fairly rapidly and felt at the mercy of something outside of myself.

I now find that I can go from low to high to low within extremely short periods of time and have been diagnosed as a "rapid, rapid" cycler or "ultradian" cycler. These constant mood fluctuations are very tiring and distressing and take a real toll on me emotionally.

12. How is bipolar disorder diagnosed?

Bipolar disorder is diagnosed as part of a complete psychiatric or other mental health evaluation. The evaluation includes a review of current and past symptoms, psychiatric and medical history, family history, social history, and substance-use history. In addition, there is an assessment of the current **mental status**. Although there are no tests or procedures to diagnose bipolar disorder, in certain circumstances tests may be ordered in addition to a request for physical examination in order to rule out any general medical conditions as a cause for the psychiatric symptoms. Depending on the circumstances, the clinician may

Mental status
snapshot portrait of one's cognitive and emotional functioning at a particular point in time. It is always included as part of a psychiatric examination.

want to obtain collateral information from family members. Based upon the symptoms, history, and mental status, a specific diagnosis can be made. The DSM-IV-TR defines six criteria sets for the diagnoses of bipolar I disorder, based upon the type of episode a person has last experienced—mania, hypomania, major depressive, or mixed.

A manic episode is defined by the following:

- Patients will have an abnormally and persistently elevated, expansive, or irritable mood lasting at least one week (or less if hospitalized), along with three or more of the following:
  a. Inflated self-esteem or **grandiosity**
  b. Decreased need for sleep
  c. More talkative than usual or pressure to keep talking
  d. **Flight of ideas** or racing thoughts
  e. Distractibility
  f. An increase in goal-directed activity or **psychomotor agitation**
  g. Excessive involvement in pleasurable activities that have a high potential for painful consequences

Symptoms of a manic episode are severe enough to cause marked functional impairment or hospitalization and are not a result of substance use or a medical condition. A **hypomanic** episode is defined by the same symptoms but is not severe enough to cause a marked impairment of functioning or hospitalization. Rather, hypomanic symptoms are a change from the afflicted individual's normal functioning and need to last at least four days. A major depressive episode is defined by the following symptoms:

Grandiosity

the tendency to consider the self or one's ideas better or more superior to what is reality.

Flight of ideas

a type of thought disorder in which there is repeated switch of topic either mid-sentence or inappropriate to the topic at hand.

Psychomotor agitation

hyperactive or restless movement. Can be seen in highly anxious states, manic mood states, or intoxicated states.

Hypomanic

milder form of mania with the same symptoms but of lesser intensity.

- Depressed mood most of the day, nearly every day, or
- Loss of interest or pleasure in activities, with four or more of the following:
  a. Significant weight loss (not from dieting) or weight gain or change in appetite
  b. Feelings of worthlessness or inappropriate guilt
  c. Decreased concentration

Hypersomnia

an inability to stay awake. Oversleeping.

  d. Insomnia or **hypersomnia** (excessive sleep)
  e. Psychomotor agitation or retardation
  f. Fatigue or loss of energy
  j. Recurrent thought of death or suicidal ideation

Again, significant functional impairment needs to be present, and symptoms can not be a result of a substance or a medical condition. A mixed episode is defined as the presence of both a major depressive and a manic episode for at least one week.

The six criteria sets for diagnosing bipolar I disorder are: single manic episode, most recent episode hypomanic, most recent episode manic, most recent episode mixed, most recent episode depressed, and most recent episode unspecified.

13. Are there different types of bipolar disorder?

Question 12 gives six criteria sets for bipolar I disorder. Other bipolar disorder diagnoses are:

- Bipolar II disorder
- Cyclothymic disorder
- Bipolar disorder not otherwise specified

Bipolar II disorder is characterized by episodes of hypomania and major depression. In contrast to bipolar I, bipolar II is diagnosed only if there is a history of both major depression and hypomania. Bipolar I can be diagnosed with a history of just mania. If there is no history of major depression, but episodes of mild depression are present, cyclothymia is diagnosed (discussed in more detail in Question 21). Bipolar disorder not otherwise specified is reserved for when there are bipolar features but full criteria are not met for another specific diagnosis. For example, bipolar disorder could be diagnosed in the presence of recurrent hypomanic episodes without a history of depression. It is also diagnosed when there is very rapid alternation of mood states that do not meet the duration criteria for each condition (one week for mania and two weeks for major depression).

In addition to the types of bipolar disorder, there are also qualifiers for the bipolar I and bipolar II diagnoses. The rapid cycling qualifier is given when there are more than four episodes of a manic, hypomanic, major depressive, or mixed episode in a one-year period. Other qualifiers are used to describe the severity of the episode, presence or absence of psychosis, postpartum onset, the longitudinal course, and stage of remission.

14. Are there any blood tests or other tests for bipolar disorder?

No objective tests are available for the diagnosis of bipolar disorder. Some tests such as blood tests or brain scans measure levels of certain chemicals or look at brain functioning. These are research based only and presently have no diagnostic utility for clinical practice. Your doctor may order blood tests to check for any underlying conditions that may mimic depression or mania. Blood tests or electrocardio-grams may be ordered for baseline purposes, depending on the medication that is to be prescribed, as some medications may have effects on certain organ systems in the body; for example, lithium may have effects on thyroid or kidney function. In addition, there is typically some level of blood monitoring over the course of treatment with many agents used in bipolar disorder.

Although rating scales and self-report forms are not a required part of an evaluation, some clinicians will use them to assist in the evaluation process. Scales may be useful in tracking the progression of symptoms in a quantifiable way. Comprehensive diagnostic scales can guide the clinician in going through a differential diagnostic process in order to exclude other causes for the symptoms before establishing a diagnosis. Such scales may indeed establish a diagnosis, but they are based on the same clinical criteria used without a scale. These scales are mostly useful in research to establish reliability in diagnosis and to improve the validity of the study.

Leslie's comments:

Frankly, I wish there were biological tests. I think having undisputed scientific evidence would "normalize" the disorder and would limit the amount of stigma people feel. It would be viewed as just another medical illness that one grapples with and I think those with the disorder would be far less hesitant to share if it were taken out of the realm of a "mental" illness.

Diagnosis

15. I can't sleep and have racing thoughts. I thought I was just really anxious, but now wonder, could I have bipolar disorder?

Many symptoms people experience occur in a variety of conditions described in the DSM-IV-TR. *Anxiety* is a term that connotes a feeling of psychic discomfort. It often includes a sense of fear of impending doom that may or may not accompany a clear sense of its source and feels out of proportion to whatever is causing the anxiety. There are several types of anxiety disorders: panic disorder, agoraphobia, specific phobia, social phobia, obsessive-compulsive disorder, posttraumatic stress disorder, acute stress disorder, and generalized anxiety disorder. Anxiety disorders may be associated with physical symptoms along with psychological discomfort. When the physical discomfort becomes extreme, anxiety is often referred to as panic. Physical symptoms associated with panic include shortness of breath, light-headedness, numbness and tingling (**paresthesias**), chest pain, palpitations, stomach upset, and diarrhea. Psychological symptoms are more difficult to characterize, but they include such feelings as worry, fear, **dysphoria**, distress, and agitation or irritability, along with a sense of impending doom. Distressing thoughts often go along with those feelings. The thoughts usually center on whatever the worrisome issue is, such as deadlines for accomplishing tasks, concerns regarding performance, and fears of impending bad outcomes resulting from recent decisions (such as financial, personal, health, or career ruin). Some of these fears can be reality based though they are usually grossly distorted. The worries are

Paresthesias

presence of numbness and tingling in limbs. Often a symptom in anxiety disorders.

Dysphoria

an emotional state of feeling unhappy or unwell.

often ruminative in nature and can be quite distracting. They are particularly bothersome when the mind is unfocused, which occurs most often at night when trying to fall asleep. These nagging worries often snowball into other worries at that point in time, leading to insomnia and the subjective feeling that one's thoughts are racing. This can in turn lead to physical agitation and hyperactivity. One can have a short fuse from lack of sleep and lowered frustration tolerance, leading to frequent arguments with others. When comparing the symptoms of some anxiety states with manic states one is immediately struck by a number of similarities—insomnia, "racing thoughts," irritability, distractibility, and lowered frustration tolerance. What looks like hyperactivity to others may actually be a subjective feeling of restlessness. Anxiety and mania both can be precipitated by stress. Although stress can be an ill-defined concept, everyone can appreciate what it means when a stressful life event occurs. Most initial reactions to stress are accompanied by anxious and irritable feelings.

Anxiety and mania have some important differences, however. Mania can be associated with predominant irritability, but it is more typically experienced as euphoria with the irritability occurring when one feels that his or her goals are being frustrated by others. Anxiety, on the other hand, is distinctly dysphoric. The nature of insomnia in the two disorders is also different. Manic patients just don't feel they need to sleep, nor do they want to sleep. They are certainly not distressed by their lack of sleep. In fact, they have too many things they need to accomplish to worry about getting sleep. Additionally, their racing thoughts are not unwanted or distressing but instead filled with wonderful ideas of things to accomplish. Their thoughts are generally **ego-syntonic**. Those with anxiety, alternatively, desperately seek sleep in order to escape their thoughts and worries. They want their minds to turn off and plead for something to stop their racing thoughts because such thoughts are psychologically painful, or **ego-dystonic**. As a result, although patients with anxiety may appear hyperactive and agitated, they subjectively feel exhausted and greatly desire escape from their feelings in the form of sound, uninterrupted sleep.

Clinical studies have also demonstrated high **comorbidity** between bipolar disorder and panic disorder, obsessive-compulsive disorder, social phobia, and post-traumatic stress disorder. In a recent study, more than half of bipolar patients had a comorbid anxiety disorder. Those with the combination of the two conditions usually had a younger age of onset, functioned more poorly, and had a greater likelihood of attempting suicide, in addition to having a poorer chance of **recovery**. Increasingly, evidence is demonstrating that anxiety associated with any psychiatric condition increases the risk of attempting suicide severalfold. Thus it is critical to have anxiety properly treated in addition to the mood instability.

Psychobiological mechanisms that may account for these high comorbidity rates likely involve a complicated interplay among various neurotransmitter systems and their response to environmental stimuli that are perceived by the organism. These neurotransmitter systems include norepinephrine, dopamine, gamma-aminobutyric acid (GABA), and serotonin. Moreover, certain antimanic medications clearly have antipanic

Diagnosis

Ego-syntonic
that which is acceptable to the self (ego).

Ego-dystonic
that which is unacceptable to the self (ego).

Comorbidity
the presence of two or more mental disorders, such as depression and anxiety.

Recovery
achievement of baseline, premorbid functioning after successful treatment for a mental illness. *Recovery* is the term used after a time period of six months symptom free. Up to that point the term used is *remission*.

Anxiolytic

a substance that relieves subjective and objective symptoms of anxiety.

Antipsychotic

a drug that treats psychotic symptoms, such as hallucinations, delusions, and thought disorders. Antipsychotics can be used to treat certain mood disorders as well.

properties and may have **anxiolytic** or anti-anxiety properties as well (e.g., Equetro (carbamazepine), Depakote (sodium valproate), and possibly **antipsychotics**). Some anxiolytics (e.g., gabapentin and benzodiazepines other than alprazolam) as well can be particularly useful in treating acute mania in bipolar patients who also suffer from anxiety.

16. What is the difference between bipolar disorder, schizophrenia, and schizoaffective disorder?

Strictly speaking, bipolar disorder is classified as a mood disorder and schizophrenia as a psychotic disorder. Schizoaffective disorder is considered primarily a psychotic disorder, but with a concurrent mood disorder. All three conditions may be diagnosed in one individual over the course of his or her illness at different points in time because of the overlap of many of the symptoms. For many disorders listed in the DSM-IV-TR, there is an overlap of symptoms, and many conditions can be diagnosed concurrently (e.g., a depressive disorder and an anxiety disorder), which is known as comorbidity. Although there are many conditions that people can have simultaneously, some conditions have as a criterion a specific exclusion of the concurrent diagnosis of another condition. Historically, individuals who have actually suffered from bipolar disorder have sometimes been inaccurately diagnosed with schizophrenia. Symptoms can be similar between these conditions, but the prognosis can be quite different, so an accurate diagnosis is important. The treatment was once vastly different, but with the advent of atypical antipsychotics, treatment options often overlap as well, so medication history is not an adequate means for determining a person's past psychiatric diagnoses.

Despite the overlap in symptoms, particularly for the manic episode of bipolar disorder, the three conditions in question cannot be diagnosed concurrently, according to the DSM-IV-TR. The symptoms for schizophrenia include the following:

- Delusions
- Hallucinations
- Disorganized speech
- Disorganized behavior
- Negative symptoms (**affective flattening**, **alogia**, **avolition**)

Any of these symptoms can be present if psychotic during a manic episode. As such, to diagnose schizophrenia, there must be the exclusion of either schizoaffective disorder or a mood disorder (such as bipolar disorder) with psychotic features. Schizoaffective disorder is defined by the presence of a major depressive or manic episode (or mixed) (see Question 12) concurrent with symptoms of schizophrenia as noted above. In addition, there needs to have been at least a two-week period of delusions or hallucinations *in the absence of* prominent mood symptoms. Thus, schizoaffective disorder often is more easily diagnosed over the course of an illness rather than at a specific point in time. An accurate history would certainly be needed to do so, and this can often be difficult to obtain, especially during an acute phase of any of these illnesses.

17. I feel happy and productive. How can I have a mental disorder?

There are several possible answers. First, you have no mental disorder and someone is over-pathologizing your upbeat, get-up-and-go attitude. The line dividing

Affective flattening
a dulling of one's facial and emotional response to external stimuli.

Alogia
the inability to speak due to mental incapacity.

Avolition
a psychological state characterized by a general lack of desire, motivation, and persistence.

normal variation in mood and pathological variation is often in the eye of the beholder. Although clinicians can generally agree on severe diagnoses like schizophrenia, bipolar I disorder, and major depressive disorder, milder variations on these disorders cast very wide nets that overlap with normal variations in personality. This is especially true for other mood disorders such as bipolar II disorder, cyclothymia, bipolar disorder NOS, depressive disorder NOS, and dysthymia. The DSM-IV-TR offers specific criteria for each of these conditions. Deciding whether a patient's particular behavior, feeling, thought or attitude represents any one of those specific criteria, however, is more subjective impression than objective application. There are also many conditions described in the scientific literature known as bipolar variants or bipolar spectrum disorders that include ultra-rapid cycling or ultradian bipolar disorder that have not yet been established by the DSM committee.

Second, what you perceive to be happy and productive may not necessarily be anything of the kind. Ask yourself whether people around you are repeatedly getting in the way of your happiness or productivity or placing obstacles in your path toward your goals. If you find that many times your claim to happiness and productivity is really just a feeling and that everyone else sees something very different, then you need to take stock of why there is such a disparity of opinion. Typically when patients are suffering from mania, they are happy but everyone around them is miserable. This is partly because when someone intrudes on a manic person's goals and happiness he or she can become extremely angry and aggressive. Irritability at this point intrudes and generally becomes the dominant mood. Manic individuals impulsively engage in reckless and hedonistic activities and do not think of the ultimate consequences of their behavior, such as bankruptcy, divorce, or worse.

Finally, the reason for your good mood may be because you are taking medication and it is working. Keep in mind that bipolar disorder is a chronic, recurrent condition and medication merely controls the symptoms and prevents **relapse**. Too often, after responding to medication, a person believes the problem is over and medication is no longer necessary. This is especially true early in treatment when one believes it was a one-time, stress-related incident that precipitated the mood episode. Although psychiatrists cannot predict the future, the issue of future episodes is a matter of evaluating the risk of relapse while off medication versus the risk of side effects while on the medication. Generally speaking, the risk of developing a clinically significant depressive episode far exceeds a relapse into mania, and it is usually the depressive episodes of bipolar disorder that are most debilitating.

Relapse

the return of symptoms of a mental illness for which one is currently receiving active treatment. Relapse occurs during response to treatment or during remission of symptoms. If symptoms return after six months of successful treatment during what is termed the recovery phase, the term used is *recurrence*.

18. How does bipolar depression differ from major depression?

The symptoms of depression in bipolar disorder are the same as in major depression. In fact the depressive episode of bipolar disorder meets the same criteria outlined for a major depressive episode in the DSM-IV-TR, as described in Question 12. The differences between the illnesses have more to do with their genetics, clinical course, prognosis, and treatment. Bipolar disorder is so often missed because the depressive episodes look the same; it takes an average of eight years for the correct diagnosis of bipolar disorder to be made in a person who presents for treatment of depression. Frequently patients fail to report a history of hypomanic or manic symptoms, but clinicians may fail to recognize past manic symptoms as well. Bipolar II disorder is more likely to be missed than bipolar I due to the reduced severity of hypomanic symptoms. It is the history that is important in making an accurate diagnosis of bipolar disorder in a depressed individual. Some clinical features, however, are thought more indicative of bipolar disorder than major depression. These include a younger age of onset (< 25 years old), presence of atypical symptoms, psychotic symptoms, and comorbid substance abuse. A family history of bipolar illness is also suggestive. Other associations include multiple depressive episodes, brief duration of depressive illness, and antidepressant-induced mania or hypomania. Although none of these associations are diagnostic of bipolar depression, they can alert a clinician to watch for future manic episodes.

Although primary care physicians often diagnose cases of depression, including a bipolar depressive episode, because of the unique difficulties in treating bipolar depression, it is critical that a psychiatrist closely follow the treatment course. Treatment of bipolar depression can be difficult because the use of antidepressant therapy poses risks for a manic switch. Lithium has historically been the mainstay for bipolar depression and has been shown to reduce risk of suicide in bipolar patients, but it has numerous side effects. Recent approval was obtained for the combination of olanzapine and fluoxetine (Symbyax) specifically for bipolar depression. Anticonvulsant medications have been preferentially utilized for treatment of manic episodes. Lamotrigine has been approved for prevention of depressive **recurrences** in bipolar disorder. If a psychiatrist determines that an antidepressant is necessary, current practice is to have a mood stabilizer on board prior to initiating the antidepressant, as this may be protective of a manic switch from the antidepressant.

19. My husband is depressed and has mood swings. Could he be a manic-depressive?

Mood swings are often thought synonymous with being manic-depressive, or having bipolar disorder. The presence of "mood swings," however, is not enough to determine that a person is bipolar. Many depressed persons can have ups and downs in their mood. The distinction is important because bipolar depression is treated differently than major depression. Bipolar disorder is less frequent than major depressive disorder, occurring in approximately 1% of the population (versus ~15% for depression). It is also more closely associated with family history, and in general it is a more severe illness. Bipolar depression differs from major depression in that the individual has to have experienced at least one manic or hypomanic episode in their lifetime. Although experiencing mania or hypomania is often referred to as having "mood swings," specific criteria are used to define these mood states. Mood swings can mean many things to many people, from constant crying to episodes of irritability or anger. Manic or hypomanic episodes are strictly characterized by a decreased need for sleep (not the same as insomnia), inflated self-esteem (grandiosity), rapid and **pressured speech** (the need to keep talking), euphoric mood, and increased activity level. Duration criteria are required to make the diagnosis as well. The criteria should be closely followed because depression

Diagnosis

Recurrence

the return of symptoms of a mental illness following complete recovery, considered to have occurred following a period of six months symptom free.

Pressured speech

characterized by the need to keep speaking; it is difficult to interrupt someone with this type of speech. Commonly seen in manic or hypomanic mood states.

alone can cause irritability and anger management problems, both of which can look like "mood swings." Accurate history is needed to ensure a correct diagnosis. Once it is determined that a manic or hypomanic episode has occurred in the past, the diagnosis must reflect that as the treatment approach may be different and there are different risks associated with taking antidepressants.

20. I became irritable and agitated on my antidepressant. My doctor thinks I have become hypomanic. What does that mean?

Bipolar disorder can be diagnosed only if someone has a history of at least one manic (bipolar I) or hypomanic (bipolar II) episode. Sometimes a person's first episode of a mood disorder is that of depression, and therefore a possibility exists that a depressed individual really has bipolar disorder. The likelihood of this occurrence increases if there is a family history of bipolar disorder. If a person with depression actually has bipolar disorder, an antidepressant may trigger the onset of a hypomanic or manic mood state, which is why bipolar depressed persons usually require a mood stabilizer when taking an antidepressant.

Becoming hypomanic or even manic on an antidepressant, however, is not by itself diagnostic of bipolar disorder. These reactions can occur in non-bipolar depressed persons, although there is some debate among experts as to whether this would be characteristic of a bipolar spectrum illness (see Question 21). If you have a manic response, your doctor will want to stop the antidepressant. Further inquiry into past personal and family history will be done to be sure evidence of past hypomanic or manic episodes wasn't missed. Once the antidepressant is stopped your hypomanic or manic symptoms should resolve. If they do not, then bipolar disorder is likely present. If resolved, another antidepressant can be tried, as the manic response won't necessarily occur with another medication. If it does occur again, a mood stabilizer may be necessary in order to take an antidepressant.

21. I have been diagnosed with cyclothymia. Does that mean a quicker recovery?

Cyclothymia is a more chronic, less severe form of bipolar disorder. By chronicity, it is meant that the mood states (either depression or hypomania) are more sustained than in bipolar disorder. By severity, it is meant that the mood states are generally not associated with either vegetative symptoms (such as sleep, appetite, or energy disturbances) or psychotic symptoms (such as delusions of guilt or grandiosity). Cyclothymia is defined in the DSM-IV-TR as having over a period of two years or more (one year in children and adolescents) the presence of numerous hypomanic episodes and numerous depressive episodes that do not meet the criteria for major depressive disorder. It is the characteristic of the depressive episodes that differentiates cyclothymic disorder from bipolar II disorder (which does have major depressive episodes). Additional criteria include not having the absence of such symptoms for greater than a two-month period. Interestingly, both cyclothymia and bipolar II can be diagnosed if a major depressive episode occurs *after* the initial two-year period of illness. As with all illnesses, the symptoms cannot be due to substance use and must cause clinically significant distress or impairment in social, occupational, or other important areas of functioning.

While cyclothymia is a distinct diagnosis, it is also considered one of the bipolar variants or spectrum disorders as described by Hagop Akiskal, a prominent research psychiatrist who outlined the variants in *Psychiatric Clinics of North America*. Akiskal's schema of bipolar subtypes include the following:

- Bipolar I: full-blown mania
- Bipolar I ½: depression with protracted hypomania
- Bipolar II: depression with hypomanic episodes
- Bipolar II ½: cyclothymic disorder
- Bipolar III: hypomania due to antidepressant drugs
- Bipolar III ½: hypomania and/or depression associated with substance use
- Bipolar IV: depression associated with hyperthymic temperament

Pharmacological

pertaining to all chemicals that, when ingested, cause a physiological process to occur in the body. *Psychopharmocological* refers to those physiological processes that have direct psychological effects.

Response

referring to at least a 50% reduction but not complete cessation of all symptoms associated with a specific mental illness, such as depression.

These subtypes are increasingly receiving attention from clinicians because the concept of the bipolar spectrum is now capturing a range of behaviors typically classified under other conditions. As one can readily see, because the symptoms are considered less severe but more chronic than in bipolar disorder, the issue of quicker recovery becomes more complicated. The first question to be considered is what treatment approach to take. Depending upon the level of distress or disability you are experiencing, the illness may warrant **pharmacological** intervention. The use of medications in the management of cyclothymia has not been researched however, mainly because the pharmaceutical companies that perform the majority of drug studies focus on the more severe forms of illness because it is easier to measure outcomes in **response** to medication. Thus any medication trial for cyclothymia or any bipolar variant will be largely empirical—that is, trial and error. Second, because the symptoms tend to last longer than in bipolar disorder, psychotherapy is critical whether or not you choose pharmacological management because it will help you develop skills to deal more effectively with stressors in the environment and negative self-thoughts that may accompany mood swings. Many people suffering from cyclothymia have comorbid personality disorders, which respond better to **psychosocial** interventions than pharmacotherapy.

22. I've been diagnosed with bipolar disorder. What do I tell my family and friends?

Although there is a greater understanding in society about both bipolar disorder and unipolar depression, stigmatization continues to exist and there can be concern about what to share about the condition with your family and friends. The decision as to sharing information about your diagnosis can be fraught with more worries as to how others will perceive you than, say, if you had to inform them of an infectious disease, a heart condition, diabetes, or even cancer. As with any other illness, you have a right to your privacy in terms of disclosure. Certainly, the more you can open up about your bipolar disorder, as with any illness, to people close to you, the more support you will have in your time of need. It is reasonable to use discretion in sharing anything about yourself that is personal; the same holds true regarding bipolar disorder. Yet if you don't discuss it with people closest to you, you may be more apt to feel shame about it, and you will be inhibited in obtaining help and remaining on the treatment

Psychosocial
pertaining to environmental circumstances that can impact one's psychological well-being.

Diagnosis

plan you need. Stigmatization results when people hide shamefully behind what ails them. It is easier for people to hold on to their biases if they believe they do not know anyone with bipolar disorder, or any other mental illness. Close family and friends are more apt to be supportive than you may believe. In addition, given the chronic nature of bipolar disorder, it may become difficult to "hide" the ongoing treatment that is required. **Subsyndromal** symptoms may appear that can confuse your friends and family if they do not know what you are suffering from. Friends and family may need to be enlisted as well to help you monitor your symptoms, as it is often difficult for a person to self-identify the onset of mania. Question 92 addresses the issue of family involvement further.

Subsyndromal

exhibiting symptoms that are not severe enough to be characterized as a syndrome.

Scott's comments:

I chose not to participate in this book under a pen name. I feel that I have no more to hide than if I were diabetic or had some other condition. My grandfather was bipolar, and I'm bipolar. I take medication to stabilize my mood swings, and I'm not at all ashamed of this condition. I look at it as simply a biological reality that I have to deal with. I hope that whatever stigma is associated with bipolar disorder is quickly eliminated, as it's less a sign of weakness than strength—strength to be willing to understand what is making us behave the way we do, particularly when that behavior doesn't serve us. I tell anyone that asks—I'm bipolar. I'm medicated. Big deal.

Leslie's comments:

Being diagnosed with bipolar disorder came as a relief because I finally had a reason for all of the mood swings I had experienced since I was a teenager. However, along with the relief came a feeling of being stigmatized; both within myself as well as in society's perception of those struggling with mental illness. I had to come to terms with these feelings before I was able to share my diagnosis with my friends and family. When I was finally able to discuss the issue, I felt very vulnerable to their reactions and was probably less open than I could have been because of this. To me, it was most important for my partner to understand what I had been going through; all of the emotional ups and downs and strain that I had put on the relationship could finally be explained, however not erased. Unfortunately, I still feel shame when I discuss my bipolar disorder with my friends and family because I believe that they look at it as just an excuse rather than a viable explanation for my erratic behavior over the years.

23. Who is qualified to diagnose and treat bipolar disorder?

In general, the need for medication when diagnosed with bipolar disorder is far greater than with depression. Bipolar disorder is much more complicated to treat medically and therefore this should be your primary concern when seeking a qualified clinician. Many clinicians of various educational backgrounds are qualified to diagnose and treat bipolar disorder to varying degrees. The choice of practitioner type in part will depend on the severity of symptoms, the need for therapy, medication, or a combination of these factors. Your internist or family practice doctor can diagnose and treat bipolar disorder to a limited degree, as can a nurse practitioner. Typically they will refer you to a mental health specialist, however, because a more in-depth evaluation is warranted. Most insurance plans have participants who can provide mental health services, although sometimes the choices available on a given plan are limited. Geographical location also may dictate choice of practitioner, as there are shortages of certain clinicians (e.g., child and adolescent psychiatrists) in some areas of the United States. Also, because of the typical need for medication in bipolar disorder (in contrast to unipolar depression), a psychiatrist should be part of the treatment team. Mental health specialists who can evaluate for and take part in the treatment of bipolar disorder include:

- Social workers
- Psychologists
- Psychiatric nurse specialists or APRNs (advanced practice registered nurses)
- Psychiatrists

In seeking a mental health specialist, it is important to choose someone with proper credentials and training. Anyone can call himself or herself a psychotherapist without having specialized training or a degree. It is appropriate to ask the therapist about his or her training and background in the assessment and treatment of bipolar disorder. Credentials for the above-noted mental health specialists follow.

Social workers provide a full range of mental health services, including assessment, diagnosis, and treatment. Most social workers work in conjunction with a physician, either a primary care practitioner or a psychiatrist who can prescribe medication. They have completed undergraduate work in social work or other fields, followed by postgraduate education to obtain a master's of social work (MSW) or a doctorate degree.

An MSW is required in order to practice as a clinical social worker or to provide therapy. Most states require practicing social workers to be licensed, certified, or registered. Postgraduate education is two years, with courses in social welfare, psychology, family systems, child development, diagnosis, and child and elder abuse/neglect. During the two years of coursework, social work students participate in internships concordant with their interest. Following completion of the master's program, direct clinical supervision is usually required for a period of time, the hours of which may vary from state to state, prior to obtaining a license.

Psychologists have completed undergraduate work followed by several years of postgraduate studies in order to receive a doctorate degree (PhD or PsyD) in psychology. Graduate psychology education includes study of a variety of subjects, notably statistics, social psychology, developmental psychology, personality theory, psychological testing (paper and pencil tests to help assess personality characteristics, intelligence, learning difficulties, and evidence of psychopathology), psychotherapeutic techniques, history and philosophy of psychology, and psychopharmacology and physiological psychology. Following the coursework, a year is spent in a mental health setting providing psychotherapeutic care and psychological testing under the supervision of a senior psychologist. Psychologists must demonstrate a minimum number of hours (usually around 1,500) before they are eligible to sit for state psychology licensure exams. In Louisiana and Arizona, psychologists have earned limited prescribing privileges and work under the supervision of a psychiatrist. These two states require psychologists to complete a clinical psychopharmacology program in addition to their other postgraduate work. This may be an option for patients if there is a scarcity of psychiatrists available to prescribe medication.

Psychiatric nurse specialists have completed undergraduate work, typically in nursing, and obtain postgraduate education in nursing at the master's or doctorate level. Master's programs are two years, with coursework consisting of study in physiology, pathophysiology, psychopathology, pharmacology, psychosocial and psychotherapeutic treatment modalities, advanced nursing, and diagnosis. The training includes clinical work under supervision. Licensing and scope of practice varies from state to state.

Psychiatrists are medical doctors with specialized training in psychiatry. They have completed undergraduate work followed by four years of medical school. Medical education is grounded in basic sciences of anatomy, physiology, pharmacology, microbiology, histology, immunology, and pathology, followed by two years of clinical rotations through specialties that include medicine, surgery, pediatrics, obstetrics and gynecology, family practice, and psychiatry (as well as other elective clerkships). During this time medical students must pass two examinations toward licensure. After graduation from medical school physicians have a year of internship that includes at least four months in a primary care specialty such as medicine or pediatrics and two months of neurology. Following internship, physicians must take and pass a third exam toward licensure in order to be eligible for licensure (and subsequently practice) in any state. Psychiatrists-in-training have three more years of specialty training in residency, the successful completion of which makes them eligible for board certification. Following residency, many psychiatrists pursue further training in a fellowship that can last an additional two years. Such fellowships include child and adolescent psychiatry, geriatric psychiatry, consultation-liaison psychiatry, addiction psychiatry, forensic psychiatry, and research. To become board certified, psychiatrists take both a written and an oral examination. Certain psychiatry specialties also have a board certification process. Board certification is not a requirement to practice and may not be obtained immediately upon completion of residency, although many hospitals and insurance companies do require physicians to be board certified within a specified number of years in order to treat patients.

In addition to seeking a private practitioner for mental health services, you have different choices of facilities and programs where you may obtain evaluation and treatment, in which various mental health specialists work, including community mental health centers, hospital psychiatry departments and outpatient clinics, university-affiliated programs, social service agencies, and employee assistance programs.

PART III

Risk/ Prevention/ Epidemiology

What are the risk factors for development
of bipolar disorder?

Are people from different ethnic backgrounds
more susceptible to bipolar disorder?

More . . .

24. What are the risk factors for development of bipolar disorder?

The concept of risk is a modern one. The word *risk* derives from the Italian *riscare*, meaning "to dare." Before such a concept was developed, the future could be predicted only by consulting the gods, prophets, or astrologers, and when bad things happened, they were attributed to fate. The concept of risk is therefore revolutionary, because it has allowed for forecasting in a large number of fields, including economics, finance, medicine, meteorology, and other natural and social science fields. Yet the concept grew not out of a need to answer important life or death questions but out of a desire to win at games of chance when money was at stake. Given certain known events that just occurred in the game, what are the odds for winning the game? From there, everything about predicting the future grew, and forecasting with degrees of certainty for future events of all kinds developed. Knowledge of risk gives one some power over future events so as to make the odds more favorable to one's goals. A very simple yet practical example is that while wearing seat belts does not change the odds of getting into an accident, it does change the odds of surviving one. In medicine, the knowledge of risk factors helps one to understand the odds of developing certain diseases. Remember, however, that odds, no matter how favorable or unfavorable, are still just odds with the outcome for any particular event still unknown. Just because your odds of developing lung cancer are greater if you smoke a pack of cigarettes a day does not mean that you will develop lung cancer and a nonsmoker will not. Neither Dana Reeve nor Andy Kaufman smoked and both succumbed to lung cancer.

There are risk factors that you can change and risk factors that you cannot. You cannot change the genes you inherit from your parents, but you can use the knowledge of your family history to help make choices in life to reduce other risk factors contributing to the probability of developing a particular disease. Thus, recommendations for various diagnostic tests for breast cancer, colon cancer, and heart disease vary depending on whether someone has a family history for a particular condition. With all of this in mind, the risk factors for bipolar disorder are as follows:

- Gender: Bipolar I occurs equally in both sexes; rapid-cycling bipolar disorder (four or more episodes a year) and bipolar II are more common in women than in men.
- Age: The age of onset of bipolar disorder varies. The age range for both bipolar I and II disorders is from childhood to 50 years, with a mean age of approximately 21 years. Most cases first present between the ages of 15 and 24. Some patients diagnosed with recurrent major depression may indeed have bipolar disorder but do not develop their first manic episode until after 50 years of age. They may have a family history of bipolar disorder. Most patients who experience their first manic episode after the age of 50 should have a full medical or neurological workup.
- Family history: **First-degree relatives** of people with bipolar I are approximately seven times more likely to develop the illness than people in the general population. Additionally, having a parent with bipolar disorder increases the odds of having another major psychiatric disorder by 50%. Twin studies demonstrate a **concordance** of 33–90% for

First-degree relative

immediate biologically related family member, such as biological parents or full siblings.

Concordance

in genetics, similarity in a twin pair with respect to presence or absence of illness.

Adoption study

a scientific study designed to control for genetic relatedness and environmental influences by comparing siblings adopted apart.

Postpartum

referring to events occurring within a specified time after giving birth. Usually within the first four weeks.

bipolar I in identical twins. **Adoption studies** prove that children whose biologic parents have either bipolar I or a major depressive disorder remain at increased risk of developing a mood disorder whether or not their adoptive parents suffer from a mood disorder as well.

- **Postpartum:** As many as half of women with bipolar spectrum illness experience an episode of depression, mania, or mixed state in the postpartum period. Bipolar disorder may have its first onset in the postpartum period as well.

- Stressful life events: A manic cycle is often either directly or indirectly linked to external stressors. Often the first sign of trouble is loss of sleep due to the increased stress leading to increased worry. The stress need not be negative. An upcoming wedding, the birth of a child, a job promotion, or other celebratory event can also lead to mania or depression.

- Premorbid personality factors: A possible association exists, particularly in patients who are cyclothymic.

- Substance abuse or alcoholism history: An association exists.

- Socioeconomic status: A possible association exists.

In bipolar disorder, the risk factors that one has control over are very limited when compared with a disease like heart disease, which has opportunities for lowering cholesterol, blood pressure, and weight through various options, including diet, exercise, smoking cessation, and prescription medications. It is often difficult, if not impossible, to change exposure to any of the risk factors for bipolar disorder mentioned here, except for substance abuse and alcoholism, and yet the perceived level of control over developing bipolar disorder is much greater than for other diseases, another paradox of mental illness! Regarding the risk of recurrence, some control over risk factors can be taken by ensuring aggressive treatment with a competent clinician or team of clinicians and sticking to the treatment plan, with frequent follow-up visits to ensure that the symptoms are controlled effectively with all available therapies. Aside from staying on medication, ensuring a regular and healthy sleep pattern will go far toward maintaining a stable mood.

25. Are people from different ethnic backgrounds more susceptible to bipolar disorder?

The concept of medicine being guided by ethnic or racial differences has recently ignited controversy over the FDA's approval of BiDil in the treatment of heart failure in blacks. The concept raises the specter of eugenics and the shortsighted notion that specific diseases exist in groups because of skin color or ethnic background. Clearly, genetic differences do exist based on so-called racial or ethnic backgrounds through the process known as assortative mating (like is attracted to and mates with like), thereby increasing the percentage of particular genes in a population that may increase one's chances for a specific disease. But this does not provide for the fact that genetic variation crosses boundaries. Just because one's skin color is different from another's does not necessarily mean he or she is susceptible to or immune from a specific disease. For example, although sickle cell anemia is usually associated with African Americans, whites can develop it as well. The color of one's skin or one's geographical origin remains only a "rough guide" in determining the odds of developing a particular disease until genetic testing becomes cheaper and easier to perform.

That being said, with respect to bipolar disorder no racial predilection exists. However, because of preconceived notions of race it is thought that populations of African Americans and Hispanics are more likely to be diagnosed with schizophrenia than with mood disorders or specifically bipolar disorder. Studies of ethnicity and bipolar disorder have found that African American groups are significantly less likely to have experienced a depressive episode before onset of first mania compared with white European groups. Research has also shown that African Americans and Hispanics experience more severe psychotic symptoms at first mania, but no differences were found in **mood-incongruent** psychotic symptoms (psychotic symptoms that do not reflect the patient's mood, such as a patient reporting grandiose delusions in the face of depression) between ethnic groups. Because acute mania can be clinically indistinguishable from acute schizophrenia, these findings may account for why these groups are diagnosed more often with schizophrenia while whites are diagnosed more often with bipolar I disorder. Whether these differences are due to some underlying genetic or environmental issue remains to be determined. If anything, because bipolar I disorder knows no real distinction between race, creed, or color, these findings lend further support to the contention that this condition is more strongly rooted in human biology than its counterpart, depression.

Mood-incongruent

symptoms that are inconsistent with the dominant mood state, such as euphoria in the presence of paranoia of being harmed.

26. I have recently been diagnosed with bipolar disorder. What are the risks my children will inherit it?

The lifelong prevalence worldwide is anywhere from 0.3 to 1.6% for bipolar I disorder and larger for bipolar II disorder, with rates adding an additional 0.5 to 4% to the total number, depending on the epidemiological study. Thus, regardless of one's background, this is the risk for the development of the disorder. Now, supposing you have the diagnosis of bipolar disorder, how much greater is the risk to your child? We know that bipolar disorder, especially bipolar I disorder, has a major genetic component, with evidence coming from several studies. First-degree relatives—that is, immediate family members who share 50% of your genes (siblings and children)—are around seven times more likely to develop bipolar I disorder than the general population. Additionally, the offspring of a parent suffering from bipolar disorder have a 50% chance of having another psychiatric disorder, independent of their chances of having bipolar disorder. Identical twin studies demonstrate a concordance rate of 33% to 90%, depending on the study. That is, if you have bipolar disorder, the likelihood of your identical twin having the disorder is between 33% and 90%. For non-identical twins, the concordance rate is between 15% and 20%. For first-degree relatives—that is, brothers and sisters who are not twins or children of parents who suffer from the disorder—the concordance rate is between 5% and 10%. Adoption studies demonstrate that the risks of developing bipolar disorder follow those of the biological parent and not the adoptive parent. Schizophrenic, schizoaffective, and manic syndromes appear to share genetic risk factors, suggesting that bipolar I disorder is more akin to a psychotic disorder than a mood disorder.

The fact that there is not 100% concordance between identical twins demonstrates, however, that environmental influences still have a role in the development of the disorder. Environmental effects can mean anything non-genetic, from local chemical environmental effects on the gene, to more global biological effects like fetal exposure to some as yet unidentified substance, to what are more commonly thought of as environmental factors such as family and social circumstances. If a patient has negative family and social circumstances, environment is considered more of a trigger than an actual cause, and any genetic vulnerability may be either protected by a stable environment or, more typically, provoked or precipitated by an unstable environment. Putting together genetic and environmental factors as contributors to the onset of bipolar disorder means that with a family history, an individual has a higher **relative risk** than anyone in the general population for developing bipolar disorder. Stressful life events, specific environmental circumstances, or certain psychological processes may serve as a trigger of a manic episode in someone with a genetic predisposition for the disorder.

Relative risk

a ratio of incidence of a disorder in persons exposed to a risk factor to the incidence of a disorder in persons not exposed to the same risk factor.

27. Is there a link between epilepsy and bipolar disorder?

Questions about a possible link between epilepsy and bipolar disorder naturally arise due to the fact that anticonvulsants also treat bipolar disorder. From a historical standpoint epilepsy was first thought to be a purely mental or psychological disease, although at that time neurologists were the only specialists who treated both neurological as well as psychiatric conditions, and most medical people felt that psychiatric disorders were fundamentally neurological in origin. Toward the end of the nineteenth century, epilepsy was beginning to be regarded as a distinct phenomenon, and controversy developed as to whether hysteria, a psychological condition, was actually due to epilepsy or to childhood trauma. Jean-Martin Charcot, a prominent neurologist in France, weighed in on the side of epilepsy, though he was most famous for his studies on hysteria utilizing hypnotism. His clinical picture of hypnotism was similar to the clinical picture he had previously developed for epilepsy. He believed that hypnotism demonstrated that hysteria was a form of epilepsy because it presented with the three clinical stages of **catalepsy**, lethargy, and **somnambulism**. Catalepsy is a type of sudden paralysis, and somnambulism is sleepwalking. Another neurologist, Sigmund Freud, who first began developing his theory of hysteria as having roots in childhood, disagreed. Ultimately Freud's arguments carried the day. Although Freud and Charcot both believed that all mental diseases were brain diseases, Freud's writings ultimately led to the development of psychotherapy for all mental illnesses and the brief historical abandonment of biological causes of mental illness.

Research has increasingly demonstrated that the incidence of neurobehavioral disorders is higher in patients with epilepsy than in the general population.

Catalepsy

a condition that occurs in a variety of physical and psychological disorders and is characterized by lack of response to external stimuli and by muscular rigidity, so that the limbs remain in whatever position they are placed.

Somnambulism

sleepwalking.

The link between neurobehavioral disorders and a particular type of epilepsy known as temporal lobe or complex partial seizures is particularly strong.

The underlying mechanisms or causes of bipolar disorder share many similarities with epilepsy. As in epilepsy, the more episodes that occur in a bipolar disorder patient early in the course of the disease, the more frequent and severe later episodes will be. This is thought to be due to a well-known phenomenon called **kindling**. Kindling is defined as seizures provoked by repeated stimulation of the brain that require less and less intensity. In animal studies a particular stimulus that once required great intensity can thus be extremely faint after kindling to provoke the same level of seizure. The seizure threshold is then considerably reduced. Kindling may also explain why the levels of stress that can precipitate a manic episode in a particular individual often become reduced over time. Additionally, anticonvulsant agents play an important role in the treatment of bipolar disorder. They affect the same neurotransmitter systems thought to play a role in both conditions—namely, the GABA/glutamate neurotransmitter systems. GABA is the brain's major inhibitory neuron, suppressing or dampening brain activity through nerve cell membrane stabilization. Glutamate is the major excitatory neurotransmitter serving to activate brain activity. Seizures can then occur by relative decreases in GABA or increases in glutamate causing large segments of neurons to fire asynchronously or haphazardly. This leads to not only motor disturbances but sensory and mental disturbances as well.

Kindling

changes that occur in the brain as a result of repeated intermittent exposure to a subthreshold electrical or chemical stimulus (such as in seizures) so that there develops a permanent decrease in the threshold of excitability.

28. I have recently been diagnosed with depression, but I have a family history of bipolar disorder. What is my risk of becoming manic if I take antidepressant medication?

Part of a comprehensive mental health evaluation involves a detailed past personal psychiatric history as well as a family psychiatric history. The family psychiatric history is important because many psychiatric conditions have a heritable component and can inform the clinician as to risks for certain conditions. Although bipolar disorder is known to have genetic links, a family history of bipolar disorder does not automatically rule in bipolar disorder in a person presenting with a major depressive episode. In the absence of a personal past psychiatric history of mania or hypomania, bipolar disorder is not diagnosed. That said, bipolar disorder can present with depression first and must always be considered even in the absence of family history of bipolar disorder. The presence of bipolar disorder in the family history increases the risk for the condition in a given individual (see Question 26), and it also increases the risk for mood disorders in general—not only bipolar disorder. In addition, the risk level needs to be kept in perspective. Although there are known heritable conditions that are either dominant or recessive, and present with a very specific risk (e.g., 50% chance of Huntington's chorea being acquired if one parent is afflicted), the risk for developing bipolar disorder, let alone any mood disorder, cannot be so precisely defined.

In such a situation, the risk of taking antidepressant medication has to be balanced against the risk of not taking it. In the case of moderate to severe depression, the risk of not taking the medication can include suicide, in addition to the consequences of significant functional impairment at work, home, and so forth. Such a risk would likely outweigh the risk for becoming manic and thus would warrant an antidepressant trial. This situation would, of course, especially require very close follow-up with a psychiatrist and may warrant that certain safeguards are put in place (e.g., a family member could monitor for signs of mania, with a specific plan for such an occurrence). As with a documented history of mania or hypomania, the psychiatrist may consider use of a mood stabilizer in conjunction with an antidepressant; however, the side effects and risks of taking a mood stabilizer, when in fact it may not be necessary, likely do not outweigh the risk for becoming manic on an antidepressant. Discuss the variables involved with your psychiatrist.

29. I have been treated for bipolar depression in the past. Can I prevent an episode in the future?

The likelihood of an individual with bipolar depression having another episode of depression as opposed to a manic episode is very high, just as the likelihood of a bipolar individual with a recent manic episode is at greater risk for the next episode being mania. In the majority of bipolar II patients, for every day spent hypomanic they will spend, on average, thirty-seven days depressed. More than half of people who have been depressed will have another episode at some point in the future. The risk for future episodes increases with more episodes of depression. The single biggest measure you can take to prevent a future episode is to stay on medication rather than to stop it. Other ways to lower the risk for recurrence include reducing stress levels and developing problem-solving strategies. Exercise, good nutrition, and adequate sleep promote a healthy sense of wellness, which can ward off negative effects of stress. In addition, a lack of adequate sleep can be associated with increased irritability, malaise, and poor functioning during the day, which may precipitate either mania or depression in someone who is vulnerable. Some people find that the use of relaxation techniques such as meditation or yoga reduces stress levels. Psychotherapy helps an individual develop new coping styles and insights into his or her responses to stressful events. Increased self-awareness and self-esteem provide reduced vulnerability to situations that could precipitate an episode. Also, early recognition of the signs and symptoms of either mania or depression allows for early treatment intervention, which can hasten recovery. The single most important recommendation, however, is to stay on your medication and seek help as soon as possible when you perceive yourself slipping back into depression so that your medication can be reevaluated.

Leslie's comments:

Experiencing bipolar depression is devastating and I live in fear that I will have another episode. In order to prevent it I stay on my medication and see a psychotherapist every week but there are times when even with these measures in place that I seem to begin slipping into a depression. I am very frightened by it and it is difficult to even go to work during these times. I begin questioning my medication; I begin questioning my purpose in life; I question whether

I'll ever feel better again. And that's not even a full-blown depression; that's just dipping my toe into that darkness.

30. What is my risk for bipolar disorder if diagnosed with cyclothymia?

Considered a less-severe form of bipolar disorder, cyclothymia is characterized by swings between hypomanic episodes and short periods of depression (that do not meet the criteria for major depression). The prevalence of cyclothymia is between 0.4% and 1% of the U.S. population, usually starting in adolescence or young adulthood. Although the presence of cyclothymia does not mean you have "early" bipolar disorder or will definitely get bipolar disorder, your risk for developing the disorder is anywhere between 15% and 50%. More importantly, the condition must be recognized when seeking treatment, as pharmacologic treatment with an antidepressant for the depressive periods can result in a switch to mania, thus making the onset of bipolar disorder more likely. If you need medication, your doctor will likely prescribe a mood stabilizer, in accordance with the guidelines for treatment of bipolar disorder. Psychotherapy can possibly reduce the risk for major depression and mania, much in the way it is used to reduce risk for relapse in bipolar disorder (Question 36).

31. Is it true that people with creative or artistic minds are at greater risk for bipolar disorder?

Probably the most well-known case of artistic genius associated with mental illness is that of Vincent Van

Gogh. During his lifetime the clear distinction between manic-depressive disorder (now known as bipolar disorder) and schizophrenia was not well established. Emil Kraeplin was the first clinician to clearly delineate these disorders phenomenologically. That is, he was the first to make careful observations about their different behavioral manifestations and course. Previously, the distinction between psychotic patients who made a full recovery and those who seemed to generally deteriorate over the course of their lives was thought due to disease versus an inherited condition. Although Van Gogh seemed to suffer from cyclical episodes, the question of Van Gogh's diagnosis remains speculative. Ernest Hemingway is often cited as another example of a genius who suffered from bipolar disorder, despite the fact that there is no evidence that he ever suffered from mania, other than his propensity to engage in risk-seeking behavior. Like most risk takers, he suffered from numerous concussions throughout his life. He was also a heavy drinker and began taking several prescription medications in his last two decades. His own psychiatrist, who never diagnosed him with manic depression, treated him for recurrent depression. The current DSM system has been in existence only twenty-five years; to apply it to ancient descriptions of artists' lives is not only complex but also culturally and historically misinformed. The need to believe in the link between artistic genius and madness remains a biased proposition from the start, and thus anytime an example of it shows itself people immediately believe it to be true.

What about current-day artists and current-day diagnostic categories? A 1986 study demonstrated a link

Risk/Prevention/Epidemiology

between artistic creativity and bipolar disorder among writers, showing that among a group of writers, 13% suffered from bipolar disorder as opposed to 2% of the general population, and 80% suffered from a mood disorder in general. More recently, a study by Kay Redfield Jamison of forty-seven British writers, painters, and sculptors from the Royal Academy found that 38% had been treated for bipolar disorder. Other studies have shown that artists report intense productively creative episodes followed by lows in output. Unfortunately, these studies suffer from small sample sizes and biases toward highly recognized award-winning individuals. Dr. Jamison has been reluctant to state that there is a definitive association, commenting that perhaps her own creativity was a consolation prize for her own bipolar illness.

Whether or not there is a link, the biggest concern that artists and writers have is that treatment of their illness will in turn sap their creativity. Given that most artists and writers do not have the luxury of relying on manic episodes to be at their creative best, it is doubtful that the highs and lows of bipolar disorder contribute much to one's creativity. Manic episodes may, however, negatively contribute to focus, concentration, and energy. There is no evidence that treatment will affect one's productivity. In fact, ample evidence shows that lack of treatment and continued episodes of highs and lows contribute greatly to one's morbidity and mortality, as Peter Kramer argues in his most recent book, *Against Depression*. Manic conditions may be viewed by the public in a romantic fashion as an indicator of a creative mind, but for those who suffer from such conditions, the reality is very much different. Bipolar conditions are as debilitating and painful as any other serious medical condition and must be treated as such.

32. A family member has bipolar disorder. Is there anything I can do to help?

Helping your family member seek treatment is one of the more important ways to assist, particularly when a patient is manic. Because mania is so often perceived by the affected individual as a positive experience, the likelihood of him or her pursuing treatment for it is close to zero. Even when depressed, many individuals have difficulty taking the first step of making an appointment with a mental health practitioner. Family support is critical to treatment success for these and other reasons. If the person is already in treatment, helping him or her remember the appointments and providing encouragement to stay in the treatment will be of tremendous help. Accompanying your family member to any appointments to provide feedback to the clinician can be of help, as some persons have difficulty identifying either symptoms of mania or depression in their condition. If the patient is on medication, assistance and reminders to take medication are useful, as a lack in **compliance** with medication is a common reason for relapse. If you believe that someone is suicidal, seek assistance as soon as possible. If a family member is manic, out of control, and in immediate danger to themselves or others and refuses to get assistance, call the local authorities, such as emergency medical services. EMS will generally bring your family member to be evaluated in the emergency room setting. Although this option is not always well received by the person involved, it is the best and may be the

Compliance
extent that behavior follows medical advice, such as by taking prescribed treatments. Compliance can refer to medications as well as to appointments and psychotherapy sessions.

only choice if someone is at risk for hurting others or, even more worrisome, killing himself or herself.

Leslie's comments:

I'd like to speak to this question from the perspective of what would be (and is) helpful to me. The key is understanding. However, understanding is not the same as being willing to go along for "the ride" as I move through my mood swings. Understanding means being able to identify behaviors in me that fall outside of my norm and making me aware of them so that I can evaluate my mood and decide if what I am feeling comes from "normal" life stressors or if I am having mood fluctuations that are induced by my brain chemistry.

Being kind and understanding about the reality of bipolar disorder without letting it be used as an excuse is the most helpful to me.

33. My mother appears to be hypomanic, but she refuses to see anyone. What can I do?

This situation can be very complicated for the family members of a person who appears to be suffering from hypomania. Hypomania can be difficult to recognize because although it is characterized by a change in functioning, by definition it does not cause marked distress or disability. It can make the person more difficult to work with because he or she is often less willing to listen to and follow directions from others as a result of inflated self-esteem, a situation that often leads to frequent arguments and irritability in the affected individual. But such symptoms can also be character traits that are always present, though perhaps to varying degrees rather than any dramatic change in personality. Also, because of the stigma of mental illness, many persons with mood disorders never seek treatment. Treatment avoidance may be more likely based on age (older), gender (male), or ethnic and cultural identity (mental illness has a greater stigma in many cultures). Perhaps your mother will not see a psychiatrist but will agree to meet with her primary care physician. You could accompany her to her appointment, where she might be willing to have you communicate concerns to the doctor. Making an initial appointment with a mental health practitioner on her behalf may be enough to motivate her to seek help, especially if you agree to attend the appointment as well. If, however, your mother absolutely refuses to meet with anyone, a decision needs to be made as to potential for dangerousness to self or others. For example, if suicidal ideation is suspected, local emergency personnel can be called to take the person to the emergency room. She may be angry about this, but if suicide is a possibility, the risk is worth taking. Some communities have mobile crisis units available in which a team of mental health practitioners can come to the home to evaluate your mother if you feel she is in crisis and agrees to the meeting. You can usually obtain information about home-based mental health services for persons in crisis from the community or city hospitals that sponsor such programs.

Leslie's comments:

It must be difficult when you see your loved one escalate to a hypomanic state. In my case, the only thing that gets through to me is being told (constantly) that my behavior isn't normal; that perhaps I should call my clinical nurse specialist to discuss my medication; that maybe I should see my psychotherapist for another opinion. Anyway, it's hard to hear this especially when I have spent so much time in a depression. It feels great to be completely energized; not needing much sleep, completely motivated to do anything and everything. It's really hard to acknowledge that I am over the top and need some help getting back on an even keel.

PART IV

Treatment

What are the different types of treatment
for bipolar disorder?

Does the type of bipolar disorder I have
determine the type of treatment I need?

What are the different types of talk
therapies and what do they do?

More ...

34. What are the different types of treatment for bipolar disorder?

Types of treatment for bipolar disorder fall into two broad categories: psychosocial treatment and pharmacological treatment. Within each category are many choices. Psychosocial treatments include individual therapies, group therapies, vocational services, family/couples therapies, as well as others. Further, there are different types of individual therapies, such as supportive, **insight-oriented**, or cognitive-behavioral. There are also various levels of treatment settings, ranging from private practice settings, outpatient clinic settings, day treatment or partial hospital programs, and inpatient treatment.

Pharmacological treatment involves the use of medications from various groups, such as anticonvulsants, antipsychotics, antidepressants, mood stabilizers, or anxiolytics. Psychotropic medicines are primarily used in psychiatric care for the treatment of mental disorders, including bipolar disorder. Many medications are utilized in other medical areas as well, such as the use by neurologists of antiseizure medications (anticonvulsants), which have been found to be efficacious in the treatment of bipolar disorder. Question 41 describes the medications used in bipolar disorder in more detail.

As part of an evaluation, your clinician will consider the most appropriate treatment plan for your bipolar illness. In part, the intervention will be based upon the phase of the illness, such as depressed, manic, or mixed. The first determination will be whether the illness can be managed acutely in the outpatient setting or best as an inpatient. Manic phases often require

Insight-oriented
also known as *dynamic*. A form of psychotherapy that focuses on one's developmental history, interpersonal relationships with one's family of origin, and current relationships with friends, spouses, and others.

hospitalization unless caught relatively early. For severe bipolar depression, hospitalization may also be required if there is risk for suicide. Patients in an acute mixed state are at particular risk for suicide due to the depression along with the impulsivity of mania. If deemed appropriate for outpatient stabilization, medication will likely be recommended along with psychotherapy. If a clinician other than a psychiatrist makes your diagnosis, he or she will likely refer you to a psychiatrist for medication consultation.

The type of therapy chosen for treatment can depend upon many factors such as cost, duration, or patient fit (Table 1). Psychosocial interventions commonly used for bipolar disorder are cognitive behavioral therapy, psychoeducation, family therapy, interpersonal, and interpersonal social rhythm therapy. Cognitive-behavioral therapy helps people with bipolar disorder learn to change inappropriate or negative thought patterns and behaviors associated with the illness. Psychoeducation serves to teach people with bipolar disorder about the illness and its treatment, and how to recognize signs of relapse so that early intervention can be sought before relapse occurs. Family therapy uses strategies to reduce the level of distress within the family that may either contribute to or result from the ill person's symptoms and can provide psychoeducation for the family members. Interpersonal social rhythm therapy helps people with bipolar disorder both to improve interpersonal relationships and to regularize their daily routines. Frequency of psychotherapy typically starts at once per week but may be more or less often depending on your individual needs or therapy type. Frequency may be increased around acute episodes. Family involvement is important as part of the therapy in bipolar disorder, as

Table 1

Therapy	Duration	Illness/Focus	Theory
Psychoanalytic or psycho-dynamic	few months to few years	personality disorders, coping skills	unconscious conflicts from childhood
Behavioral	6–20 sessions	anxiety disorders, depression, psychosomatic symptoms	symptom reinforcement
Cognitive	10–20 sessions	depression, obsessive-compulsive disorder	negative thoughts
Interpersonal	12 sessions	depression	relationship focused
Interpersonal social rhythm therapy	long-term	bipolar disorder	relationship and daily routine focused
Dialectical behavioral	one year or greater	borderline personality disorder	reduction of self-injurious behaviors
Psychoeducational	long-term	families of schizophrenic patients	support and education
Supportive	brief	acute grief reactions	reinforcing patient's strengths
Group	open-ended or time-limited	mood disorders, anxiety disorders, schizophrenia	support and education
Family	short to long-term	family roles, support, education, dynamics	various

family members need to be aware of and able to inform the clinician of any signs of relapse.

Again, as part of the treatment plan, the treatment setting also needs to be determined. Most individuals can be treated in private office settings or outpatient clinic settings. Sometimes, a higher level of structure is needed in which more services can be provided, on a daily basis, such as in a day treatment program. If impairments are severe, or safety is in question, hospitalization may be warranted.

35. Does the type of bipolar disorder I have determine the type of treatment I need?

The type of treatment intervention needed is going to be dependent more on the phase of illness you are in. When speaking of pharmacological treatments of bipolar disorder, usually it is bipolar I disorder that is specifically being addressed, although the same medications are utilized in bipolar II disorder. A manic individual is more likely to require hospitalization, while a hypomanic person can be managed in an outpatient setting. If psychotic symptoms are present, your clinician will more likely prescribe an antipsychotic agent. The pattern of episodes is also useful in determining what mood stabilizer is likely to be helpful. Lithium is typically most beneficial for cases considered "classic"—that is, with alternating episodes of depression and mania with euthymic mood in between. For persons with history of mania only without depressive episodes, an anticonvulsant such as Depakote (valproate) is typically prescribed. Mixed episodes or patterns of rapid cycling usually require the use of Depakote (valproate) or Equetro (carbamazepine). Atypical antipsychotics are often added to a mood stabilizer but can be prescribed alone, although often one medication is not enough, and a second agent is needed for stabilization.

Psychotherapy is a necessary part of treatment for all types of bipolar disorder, but during the manic phase it is likely to be supportive and educational only.

36. What are the different types of talk therapies and what do they do?

Following your consultation, the clinician will recommend the most appropriate treatment or therapeutic approach for your circumstances. The type of therapy that is useful in part depends on the stage of the illness. Most therapeutic approaches are going to be useful for bipolar depressive episodes, as it is optimal to be able to minimize or avoid the use of antidepressant medication because of the risk for manic switch. Most individuals are not amenable to therapy in the midst of a manic phase. Patients in this stage usually have quite limited insight, and treatment approaches typically need to be supportive and educationally focused. For bipolar depression or bipolar II disorder, there are many different approaches to consider. Many therapists utilize a combination of therapeutic approaches in their work. Some approaches are:

Psychodynamic therapy assumes symptoms, such as in depression, are due to unresolved, unconscious conflicts from childhood. It is based upon the classic psychoanalytic approach developed by Sigmund Freud. The therapist uses the concepts of **transference, countertransference**, **resistance**, free association, and dreams in order to help the patient develop insight into patterns in relationships that can then effect

Transference

the unconscious assignment of feelings and attitudes to a therapist from previous important relationships in one's life (parents and siblings).

Countertransference

the attitudes, opinions, and behaviors that a therapist attributes to his or her patient, based not on the true nature of the patient but rather on the biased nature of the therapist because the patient reminds the therapist of his or her own past.

Resistance

the tendency to avoid treatment interventions, often unconsciously (e.g., missing appointments, arriving late, forgetting medication).

change. It is a nondirective therapy. Although classic analytical therapy can last for years, with sessions four to five days per week, psychodynamic therapy may be shorter in duration, with sessions one to three times per week. Controlled research studies examining the **efficacy** of this type of therapy are minimal, due to the nature of this type of therapy. This treatment approach is often helpful for those with chronic coping difficulties or with personality disorders. This therapy approach does not address bipolar illness specifically.

Interpersonal therapy is useful for depression, conceptualizing it in a patient with the three components of symptom formation, social functioning, and personality factors. It focuses on the patient's social, or interpersonal, functioning, with expected improvement in symptoms. The goal is to improve communication skills and self-esteem. It is a brief and highly structured, manual-based psychotherapy. Areas of social functioning that may be addressed are interpersonal disputes, role transitions, grief, and interpersonal deficits. Therapy is focused and brief in duration, typically lasting twelve to sixteen sessions. Research studies have shown it to be an effective treatment for depression.

Interpersonal social rhythm therapy (IPSRT) is a relatively new treatment specifically geared toward the management of bipolar disorder, and it is based on the idea that disruptions in daily routines and problems in interpersonal relationships can cause recurrence of the manic and depressive episodes of bipolar disorder. During the treatment, therapists help patients understand how changes in daily routines and the quality of their social relationships and their social roles can affect their moods. After identifying situations that can trigger mania or depression, therapists teach the

Treatment

Efficacy
the ability to produce a desired effect, such as the performance of a drug or therapy in relieving symptoms.

Interpersonal therapy
a form of therapy. Unlike insight-oriented or dynamic therapy that focuses on developmental relationships, interpersonal therapy focuses strictly on current relationships and conflicts within them.

Interpersonal social rhythm therapy
a form of therapy based on the principles of interpersonal therapy. Specifically geared toward the treatment of bipolar disorder with monitoring of daily activities, including sleep.

individuals how to better manage stressful events and better maintain positive relationships. In bipolar illness, focusing on improvement of interpersonal relationships can be very important, as these are often adversely impacted by the illness. In addition, the therapy can be used to help regularize daily routines that can help in prevention of manic episodes.

Cognitive-behavioral therapy

a combination of cognitive and behavioral approaches in psychotherapy, during which the therapist focuses on automatic thoughts and behavior of a self-defeating quality in order to make one more conscious of them and replace them with more positive thoughts and behaviors.

Cognitive-behavioral therapy assumes that symptoms are due to a pattern of negative thinking. It works to help patients identify and change inaccurate perceptions of themselves and situations. It also is brief in duration and manual-based, typically lasting for ten to twenty sessions. It typically involves the use of homework assignments between sessions. Research studies have shown it to be an effective treatment for depression and some anxiety disorders. In bipolar illness, it can be especially helpful for bipolar depression, when use of antidepressant therapy may be deemed risky. See Question 38 for further discussion on cognitive-behavioral therapy.

Scott's comments:

I discovered after my diagnosis that I had been hiding or shielding my condition (quite well I might add) from my MFCC therapist. I have been in some form of talk therapy since 1988 and my bursts of rage were easily deflected to my wife's incessant nagging, irrational requests, or lack of sympathy for my ability to hear her due to my state of mind, work distractions, etc. I did a heck of a job keeping this out of the therapists' office. After my diagnosis, I found that cognitive behavioral therapy did little in my case to assuage the condition. If I take my medication regularly, I'm fine. If I forget, I feel the manic state come on. In my case, it's very physiological.

37. How do I choose a therapist and a therapy approach?

Choosing a therapist can be an overwhelming task. One look in the Yellow Pages shows lists of names, and not every therapist is listed there. One factor to consider is that there are many possible credentials of therapists. Some people identify themselves as therapists but do not have credentials that require licensure within their state. In general, a licensed practitioner will have been through a screening process that usually involves testing within their field. Level of training is another consideration. There are master's levels (social workers), doctorate levels (psychologists), as well as medical doctorate levels (psychiatrists) who do psychotherapy. Clinicians of various credentials may then have further training within a specific area of psychotherapy, such as psychoanalysis.

In the treatment of bipolar disorder, you will most likely need medication, thus it may be more fruitful to see a psychiatrist who also performs psychotherapy. Due to cost considerations, however, this option is not always feasible. Many insurance plans will provide reimbursement for master's level therapists only, whose fees usually are less than those of psychologists or psychiatrists. If there is a specific treatment modality in mind, one method of finding a therapist is to obtain referrals from professional societies for that specific modality. If modality is not the issue of concern, referrals can be obtained from a primary care physician. You may ask the therapist questions over the phone and arrange a consultation. If you are uncomfortable with the therapist following the consultation, it is important to consider the reasons for your discomfort. Sometimes individual psychological issues are **projected** onto the therapist immediately and thus are

Projected

the attribution of one's own unconscious thoughts and feelings to others.

Automatic thoughts

thoughts that occur spontaneously whenever a specific, common event occurs in one's life, and which are often associated with depression.

Overgeneralization

the act of taking a specific event, usually psychologically traumatic, and applying one's reactions to that event to an ever-increasing array of events that are not really in the same class but are perceived as such.

Catastrophic thinking

a type of automatic thought during which the individual quickly assumes the worst outcome for a given situation.

Schema

representations in the mind of the world that affect perception of and response to the environment.

Contingency contracting

use of reinforcers, or rewards to modify behaviors.

avoided by failing to continue to see the therapist. But certainly there needs to be a fit with the therapist's style in order to develop a working relationship.

38. What is cognitive-behavioral therapy?

Cognitive-behavioral therapy (CBT) is based upon two separate theoretical models, both cognitive and behavioral. Cognitive models are based upon the premise that cognitions, or thoughts, determine emotions and behavior. **Automatic thoughts** are one type of cognition that may be distorted by errors of thinking such as **overgeneralization**, **catastrophic thinking**, jumping to conclusions, or personalization. Errors in thinking tend to be more frequent and intense in depression as well as in other psychiatric disorders. Behavioral models are based upon theories of learning such as by modeling or by reinforcement to certain responses.

Cognitive-behavioral therapy uses techniques based upon the models described above. A greater emphasis on cognitive approaches or on behavioral approaches may be taken depending upon the disorder and the stage of treatment. Cognitive techniques include:

- Psychoeducation
- Modifying automatic thoughts
- Modifying **schemas**

Behavioral techniques include:

- Activity scheduling
- Breathing control
- **Contingency contracting**
- Desensitization/relaxation training

- Exposure and **flooding**
- Social skills training
- **Thought stopping**/distraction

Through many of these techniques, patients learn to manage their anxiety and reactions to stress appropriately. Exposure training is a technique that uses **graded exposure** to a high-anxiety situation by breaking the task into small steps that are focused on one by one.

CBT has been the best-studied form of psychotherapy, and it has been shown to effectively treat depression and thus can be a very effective treatment for acute cases of mild to moderate depression in bipolar disorder, when antidepressant exposure needs to be minimized. Treatment typically lasts three to six months with ten to twenty weekly sessions. The patient is expected to be an active participant in trying out new strategies and will be expected to do homework.

39. Are there any risks from engaging in psychotherapy?

Psychotherapy appears, on the surface, to be one of the most benign forms of medical therapies. There is (usually) no physical contact. No medications are prescribed. Only words are exchanged between people, nothing more. But never underestimate the force of words. There is a parable that may be recalled from childhood: "Sticks and stones may break my bones but names will never hurt me." Such a parable was created to provide comfort from the emotional wounds received from being called names. Words carry power. Just as psychotherapy has the power to heal, it also has

Flooding

exposure to the maximal level of anxiety as quickly as possible.

Thought stopping

a technique used to suppress repetitive thoughts.

Graded exposure

a psychotherapeutic technique applied to rid a patient of specific phobias. A gradual exposure to the phobic situation is set about first through imagery techniques, then through limited exposure in time and intensity before full exposure occurs.

Treatment

the power to harm. The various harms range from lack of progress to outright abuse. Most harm from psychotherapy comes from what are known as boundary violations between the therapist and the patient. The most obvious boundary violation stems from sexual or physical relationships that can develop between the therapist and patient. In many states this boundary violation is considered a criminal offense because the power differential between the patient and clinician is so great as to put the patient in a particularly vulnerable position.

Other boundary violations are not as obvious. Simple exchanges of personal information between the patient and therapist are often considered to be boundary violations and may or may not lead to more serious offenses on the part of the therapist. The potential dangers are that they may lead to friendly meetings that move beyond the office, and friendly meetings may turn more intimate. Many patients may experience their therapists as a friend; such feelings generated are known in therapy as transference. Transference is an artificial relationship that the patient projects onto the therapist. In insight-oriented or **dynamic** (Freudian) psychotherapy a transference relationship is intentionally created to allow the therapist to better understand a patient's outside relationships. This in turn allows the therapist to help a patient develop insight or greater understanding into the unconscious motives behind his or her relationships so that healthy interactions can be learned.

Dynamic

referring to a type of therapy that focuses on one's interpersonal relationships, developmental experiences, and the transference relationship with his or her therapist. Also known as insight-oriented.

Therapists also develop transference relationships with their patients, known as countertransference. If the therapist is unaware of his or her countertransference, then his or her behavior can reflect the therapist's own outside relationships rather than the patient's. If such relationships are problematic this in turn could be projected onto the patient. As a result a patient may be made to feel that he or she is experiencing problems that are really the problems of the therapist. Patients often idolize their therapist, which makes patients particularly vulnerable to the influence of their therapist's words.

A notable example of the vulnerability patients can have in therapy occurred a few years back when some cases were made public of patients believing through their therapists' suggestions that their parents sexually abused them. The process by which this occurred came about through the implantation of false memories on the part of their therapists. The therapists did not do this intentionally. In their zeal to associate certain symptoms their patient's presented with to a history of sexual abuse, they began to gradually convince their patients they had repressed memories of abuse. Once they had convinced their patients of past abuse, false memories could easily be constructed by asking them to imagine being abused or by implanting false memories through hypnosis. The term *false memory syndrome* was coined and several high-profile legal cases occurred in which patients sued their therapists for psychological damages as a result of the patients taking action on their false memories.

How can you reduce such risks? You must rely primarily on referrals and word of mouth from friends as well as other professionals. Generally your primary care doctor has developed relationships with various therapists over the years and knows their work. Success in therapy is not so much dependent upon the academic degree of the therapist as is the therapist's training and experience in treating patients. Secondarily, you need to maintain an open mind to make changes if uncomfortable with a particular therapist, no matter how skilled he or she may be. Chemistry between patient and therapist is needed, and no amount of training provides that for any particular patient. Success in therapy depends on how one feels about the therapy sessions as well as the motivation from the therapist to "do the work" outside of therapy in order to make the changes needed.

Leslie's comments:

It is really important to do your homework when choosing an appropriate therapist. It's easy to feel intimidated when speaking with a therapist for the first time but remember, in the simplest terms, you are a "consumer" of a "service" and therefore you need to find someone who will be a good fit for you as you do your work.

I made the mistake once of not doing enough homework. I saw a therapist for a few appointments and was made to feel like a dangerous "monster" because of my bipolar disorder; she was actually afraid of me. Needless to say, this experience did far more damage than good.

I am now in long term therapy with a licensed clinical social worker. We work very well together and she is extremely helpful as I face the challenges inherent in this disorder.

40. How is psychotherapy helpful if bipolar disorder is due to a chemical imbalance?

Every thought, feeling, and behavior is associated with a chemical change in the brain. If thoughts, feelings, and behaviors occur with a repeated pattern, structural changes can occur in the brain as well. Learning and memory involve complex chemical changes that lead to permanent structural changes in brain anatomy. For example, consider the first time that you learned how to drive a car. It required conscious processing of complex pieces of information and integrating the information into an organized behavioral pattern. The powers of concentration at that time can be exhausting. However, with practice the skill becomes second nature as the brain adapts the skill so that much of it occurs unconsciously. Behavior ultimately leads to structural and biochemical changes in the brain.

The chemistry and structure of the brain can change via one of three methods:

1. Change in the environment
2. Change in brain chemistry via chemical modification with the use of psychotropic medication
3. Learning how to modify the environment or perception of the environment by developing new skills

Moving, changing jobs, and getting married or divorced are examples of the first method, while psychopharmacology is the second. Psychotherapy is the third method. Brain imaging studies have repeatedly demonstrated, for example, that changes occur in the same brain regions of patients with obsessive-compulsive disorder on Sarafem (fluoxetine) as those receiving cognitive-behavioral therapy. Each of these methods has their own inherent costs and benefits and therefore none can be considered inherently better or worse than another. The effects of all three methods are generally cumulative; thus in order for one to have the best chance of recovery from mental illness, a combination of two to three methods is generally warranted.

In bipolar depression, therapy can be especially useful in an attempt to treat the depression without an antidepressant or with as low a dose of an antidepressant as possible. Therapy can help patients maintain daily structure and rhythm to help prevent the recurrence of mania. During a manic episode, therapy provides support and psychoeducation that are critical for treatment adherence and recovery.

41. What are the different types of medication used to treat bipolar disorder? How does my doctor choose a medicine?

The treatment of bipolar disorder is fraught with controversy. The two most controversial issues include the definition of a "mood stabilizer" and the use of antidepressant medications for the bipolar depressed patient. A true mood stabilizer should ideally treat acute mania, acute depression, and prevent both relapse and recurrence of either mania or depression. By that definition there is really no true mood stabilizer outside of electroconvulsive therapy (**ECT**), which is successful in treating all categories of bipolar illness. Typically, therefore, most clinicians equate the term *mood stabilizer* with a medication that treats acute mania and prevents its recurrence. More appropriately, these should be termed antimanic agents, as they are parallel to antidepressant agents and treat the other end of the mood spectrum. All mood stabilizers fail in the treatment of acute depression. The jury is out as to whether they prevent depression in the same way they prevent mania. For this reason antidepressants are still commonly used. But because antidepressant medications may switch an individual from depression into mania and actually worsen one's overall condition, the issue of antidepressant use remains controversial. Complicat-

ECT

electroconvulsive or shock therapy.

ing this issue is the fact that some clinicians define a mood stabilizer as any agent that treats one arm of the bipolar spectrum without causing switching to the other arm. By this definition, some antidepressants may meet this standard, though the jury is out in this regard as well. It does appear that some classes of anti-depressants cause less switching than others. These classes include the SSRIs and buproprion. Also by this definition the anticonvulsant Lamictal (lamotrigine) has been called a mood stabilizer even though it is clearly more effective in preventing a depressive relapse or recurrence than a manic relapse or recur-rence. Thus, the term *mood stabilizer* is generally used very loosely to describe any medication that treats "mood swings," an equally vague term that can mean just about any type of emotional change, even those associated with personality disorders such as border-line personality (Question 72). One final caveat: most antimanic agents stabilize neuronal cell membranes. As a result, any type of overstimulation of the central nervous system, whether it is seizure activity, mania, a panic attack, or explosive rage, can respond to an anti-manic agent. Therefore, the fact that one's mood is "stabilized" by an antimanic agent does not necessarily mean one is bipolar.

With that introduction let us now proceed with the different classes of medications that are used in the treatment of bipolar disorder. The classes more specifi-cally break down into several of the following cate-gories in order of understanding and importance in treating the condition:

- Lithium carbonate and its different formulations
- Anticonvulsant medications

- Atypical antipsychotic medications
- Typical antipsychotic medications
- **Benzodiazepines**
- Antidepressant medications (specifically the selective serotonin reuptake inhibitors, or SSRIs)
- Calcium channel blockers
- Mood stabilizers
- Others under investigation

Benzodiazepine

a drug that is part of a class of medication with sedative and anxiolytic effects. Drugs in this class share a common chemical structure and mechanism of action.

Note that the antimanic effects of anticonvulsants do not exhibit a class effect. That is, just because a medication is considered an anticonvulsant one cannot immediately assume it has antimanic properties. This was prominently demonstrated after the medication Neurontin (gabapentin) was touted for its potential antimanic effects prior to any clinical trials, which later demonstrated that it was not superior to **placebo** and led to a series of lawsuits against the manufacturer for false promotion. Alternatively, both the typical and atypical antipsychotics all demonstrate antimanic effectiveness and therefore clearly exhibit a class effect.

Placebo

an inert substance that when ingested causes absolutely no physiological process to occur but may have psychological effects.

Table 2 lists the specific medications, whether or not FDA approved, whether or not clinical trials exist to demonstrate their effectiveness, and whether or not they are routinely used clinically regardless of either FDA approval or the existence of clinical trials supporting their use. Bear in mind that this table does not represent all the medications used to treat bipolar disorder but rather the most common. The majority of medications used in the treatment for bipolar are used **off-label** as they are not FDA approved. First, the FDA is slow to approve medications. Second, pharmaceutical companies are slow to perform clinical trials.

Off-label

prescribing of a medication for indications other than those outlined by the Food and Drug Administration (FDA).

Trials are expensive, and once a drug is approved for acute mania, the need to seek approval for the other aspects of the condition diminishes considerably unless increase in market share can be anticipated with FDA approval. Third, once a drug becomes generic, only the government will spend money on a clinical trial. Finally, just because there are negative clinical trials does not mean that a medication is no longer used. There is enough individual variability in bipolar disorder to not immediately discount any medication, particularly when one is refractory to those medications that have proven beneficial. This is one reason why Neurontin (gabapentin) continues to be used, although in a very limited, circumscribed manner today than prior to the uproar around it. There are individuals who may idiosyncratically respond to one medication just as there are individuals who have idiosyncratic paradoxical responses to another, neither of which condition can be predicted.

Although Table 2 looks complicated, there are published treatment guidelines and algorithms that psychiatrists follow in order to simplify this table and start with the most appropriate medication depending upon the clinical presentation. There also appear to be many differences between bipolar I and bipolar II disorder. All clinical trials leading to FDA approval are based on bipolar I disorder, and it is not clear if these medications have the same effect on bipolar II disorder. It is also not clear if bipolar II disorder is truly a "spectrum" disorder—that is, lying on a continuum with bipolar I disorder rather than a unique entity itself. This uncertainty is partly based on genetic studies that suggest that bipolar I disorder shares more genes in

Table 2 Medications utilized in the treatment of bipolar disorder

Medication	Acute mania	Acute depression	Prevention of mania	Prevention of depression	Notes
Lithium Carbonate	Y, B, C	N, U, C	Y, B, C	N, L, C	Very mild antidepressant; better antimanic; prevents suicide
Valproate	Y, B, C	N, NB, NC	N, L, C	N, U, C	Anticonvulsant; better for dual diagnosis
Carbamazepine†	Y, B, C	N, L, C	N, L, C	N, L, C	Anticonvulsant; best for rapid cycling
Oxcarbamazepine	N, U, C	N, U, NC	N, U, C	N, U, C	Anticonvulsant; variant of carbamazepine
Lamotrigine	N, U, NC	N, U, C	Y, L, C	Y, B, C	Anticonvulsant; only other agent approved for bipolar depression; poor antimanic
Gabapentin	N, NB, C	N, U, NC	N, NB, C	N, U, NC	Anticonvulsant; lawsuit for promoting off-label with negative studies of benefit
Tiagabine	N, U, C	N, U, NC	N, U, C	N, U, C	Anticonvulsant; new agent; affects GABA
Topiramate	N, NC	N, NC	N, U, C	N, U, NC	Anticonvulsant; best as adjunct for weight loss
Quetiapine	Y, B, C	Y, B, C	N, U, C	N, U, C	Atypical; recent study (+) in depression
Clozapine	N, B, C	N, U, NC	N, L, C	N, U, NC	Atypical; gold standard antipsychotic; prevents suicide; weight gain; increased lipids, glucose
Olanzapine	Y, B, C	N, U, C	Y, L, C	Y‡, U, C	Atypical; weight gain; increased lipids, glucose
Olanzapine/ Fluoxetine	N, U, NC	Y, B, C	N, L, C	N, L, C	Atypical/SSRI combination; first approved drug in bipolar depression
Risperidone	Y, B, C	N, U, NC	N, L, C	N, U, C	Atypical; only agent available as long-term injectable
Ziprasidone	Y, B, C	N, U, C	N, L, C	N, L, C	Atypical; has potential SSRI-like chemical properties
Aripiprazole	Y, B, C	N, U, NC	Y, B, C	Y‡, L, C	Atypical; unique dopamine partial agonist

Table 2 Medications utilized in the treatment of bipolar disorder (continued)

Medication	Acute mania	Acute depression	Prevention of mania	Prevention of depression	Notes
Haloperidol	N, B, C	N, U, NC	N, L, C	N, U, NC	Typical; the granddaddy of acute antimanic agents
Perphenazine	N, B, C	N, U, NC	N, L, C	N, U, NC	Typical; recently compared w/atypicals in schizophrenia
Clonazepam	N, L, C	N, U, C	N, U, C	N, U, C	Benzodiazepine, anticonvulsant properties
Lorazepam	N, L, C	N, U, C	N, U, C	N, U, C	Benzodiazepine, anticonvulsant properties
Alprazolam	N, U, C	N, L, C	N, U, C	N, U, C	Benzodiazepine, anticonvulsant properties; thought once to have antidepressant properties
Citalopram & Escitalopram	N, NB, NC	$\underline{Y}$*, B, C	N, NB, NC	N, L, C	SSRI; less or no switching compared to older antidepressants
Fluoxetine	N, NB, NC	$\underline{Y}$*, B, C	N, NB, NC	N, L, C	SSRI; less or no switching compared to older antidepressants
Sertraline	N, NB, NC	$\underline{Y}$*, B, C	N, NB, NC	N, L, C	SSRI; less or no switching compared to older antidepressants
Paroxetine	N, NB, NC	$\underline{Y}$*, B	N, NB, NC	N, L, C	SSRI; less or no switching compared to older antidepressants
Verapamil	N, U, C	N, U, NC	N, U, C	N, U, NC	Calcium channel blocker; for refractory cases

Key: $\underline{Y}$ = FDA approved; N = Not FDA approved; N = Not clinical trials; B= Beneficial/strong clinical trials; L = Likely beneficial/clinical trials supportive; U = Unknown benefit/no clinical trials; NB = No benefit/negative clinical trials; C = Clinically used; NC = Not clinically used.

*For major depression, *not* bipolar depression.

†Only XR is approved for acute mania.

‡For bipolar maintenance; time to relapse for mania or depression was reduced in clinical trials, but a specific indication for *bipolar depression* is not given. Persons enrolled in the studies had a recent mixed or manic episode.

Treatment

common with schizophrenia and schizoaffective disorder than with bipolar II disorder. It is also partly based on at least some clinical reports that bipolar II patients may respond differently to the listed medications than bipolar I patients.

That being said, the general guideline makes the following recommendations. If a patient presents with acute mania, use of one medication is indicated; the choice between lithium and Depakote (valproate) is based partly on each medication's side-effect profiles as well as the presence or absence of various symptoms. For example, for patients who have suffered from depression but are currently manic, lithium is recommended. Lithium appears to be the closest to meeting the definition of a mood stabilizer in that it appears to prevent both depression and mania. For those patients who have recurrent manic episodes without depression, anxiety/agitation, or a substance abuse disorder, valproate is recommended. Patients with rapid cycling symptoms (four or more episodes annually) may respond better to either Equetro (carbamazepine) (if the episodes include more depression) or Depakote (valproate) (if the episodes include more mania). For manic patients with psychotic features (delusions, hallucinations, and/or grossly disorganized thinking and behavior) the addition of an atypical antipsychotic medication is recommended, but most atypical antipsychotics have FDA approval for monotherapy treatment of an acute manic episode. Table 3 lists the medications with FDA approval for bipolar disorder. Alternatives to lithium and Depakote (valproate) include Equetro (carbamazepine) and Trileptal (oxcarbamazepine). If symptoms are not adequately controlled within 10 to 14 days, addition of a second first-line agent is indicated (e.g., adding an anti-

Table 3 Medications with FDA Approval for Bipolar Disorder

Atypical Antipsychotics	Anticonvulsants/Others
Risperidone (Risperdal)	Valproate (Depakote, Depakote ER)
Olanzapine (Zyprexa, Zydis)	Carbamazepine XR (Equetro)
Quetiapine (Seroquel)	Lamotrigine (Lamictal)
Ziprasidone (Geodon)	Lithium (Lithobid, Eskalith)
Aripiprazole (Abilify)	Olanzapine/fluoxetine (Symbyax)

psychotic if not already prescribed). Clozaril (clozapine) may be effective in refractory cases.

For bipolar depression, either Lamictal (lamotrigine) alone (or with an antimanic agent) or Symbyax should be initiated. If one fails to respond to these two strategies the addition of Seroquel (quetiapine) or lithium may be recommended. Failing that, an additional antimanic agent plus an SSRI, buproprion, or Effexor (venlafaxine) may be added. Electroconvulsive therapy (ECT) is considered for more refractory cases (as well as for refractory mania).

Trials of nontraditional medications such as calcium channel blockers, stimulants, or thyroid hormone should be considered in conjunction with all of the above when symptoms cannot be adequately controlled. This is known as **rational polypharmacy,** as medications from different classes with different actions are added that may have a synergistic effect to improve mood stability.

Leslie's comments:

This is difficult because each prescriber has a different theory on what makes the best combination of medication. I have been on so many different medications trying to get it

Rational polypharmacy
the practice of combination medication therapy with consideration of the clinical effects, adverse effects, drug interactions, and relation between effective and toxic drug levels, as well as with an understanding of the mechanisms of action of each agent.

"right." It can become very disheartening to try a medication, take the time to build up to a therapeutic dose, and then realize that either it's not working or the side effects cannot be tolerated. Sometimes I have felt like a guinea pig trying these medications but, in the end, it does pay off because when you find the right medications, the disorder is manageable. Right now I am on an antidepressant, a mood stabilizer, and an atypical antipsychotic. This seems to be a good combination for me.

42. What are the side effects of medication for bipolar disorder?

Side effects can occur with all medications, not just psychotropic medications. In bipolar disorder however, medications are taken for long periods, so some side effects may not be tolerable because of the duration of treatment required. Side effects vary both within a class of medications and between classes, although the group of atypical antipsychotics have more similar side-effect profiles than the group of anticonvulsants, for example. In the case of antidepressants, there are even greater similarities within groups (i.e., SSRIs versus tricyclics). Even if medications of one class share similar side effects, however, the same effect will not necessarily occur with a change to another agent in the same class.

Table 4 lists some of the common side effects for the routinely prescribed mood stabilizers, and Table 5 lists the side effects from the antidepressants by class. Some medications have rare but serious side effects as well as long-term risks (see Question 61). Your doctor should go over these with you. Some side effects can be useful in certain situations. For example, in a person who has insomnia, a more sedating medication may be helpful

Table 4 Adverse effects of medications used in the treatment of bipolar disorder

Medication	Potential Adverse Effects*
valproate/valproic acid (Depakote, Depakote ER)	abdominal pain, alopecia, anorexia, diarrhea, irregular menstrual periods, nausea, tremor, vomiting, weight gain, somnolence, blurred vision, thrombocytopenia, liver failure, pancreatitis
lithium (Lithobid, Eskalith)	tremor, excessive urination, thirst, nausea, diarrhea, sedation, urinary incontinence, acne, weight gain, hypothyroidism, renal dysfunction
carbamazepine/XR (Tegretol[†], Equetro)	dizziness, drowsiness, nausea, vomiting, bone marrow suppression, rash, hypersensitivity reactions, blurred vision, impaired cognition, hyponatremia, diarrhea
oxcarbamazepine (Trileptal)[†]	abdominal pain, blurred vision, dizziness, fatigue, tremor, headache, nausea, vomiting
lamotrigine (Lamictal)	blurred vision, dizziness, sedation, nausea, anxiety, rash, tremor, blood dyscrasias, Stevens-Johnson syndrome
tiagabine (Gabitril)[†]	chills, diarrhea, impaired concentration, dizziness, bruising, fever, depression, seizure (off-label usage in nonepilepsy patients has resulted in onset of seizure disorder)
topiramate (Topamax)[†]	amnesia, impaired concentration, diarrhea, blurred vision, impaired cognition, fatigue, weakness, irregular menstrual periods, gait disturbance, anxiety, mood problems, metabolic acidosis, liver failure, pancreatitis
gabapentin (Neurontin)[†]	blurred vision, dizziness, sedation, dyskinesia, nystagmus, edema, tremors, visual changes, mood changes
olanzapine/fluoxetine (Symbyax)	side effect profile of olanzapine plus anxiety, diarrhea, insomnia, nausea, headache, sexual dysfunction
clozapine (Clozaril)[†]	constipation, dizziness, sedation, fever, nausea, sialorrhea, weight gain, arrhythmia, agranulocytosis, blood dyscrasias
risperidone (Risperdal)	agitation, sedation, headache, dizziness, constipation, diarrhea, rhinitis, blurred vision, akathisia, extrapyramidal symptoms, weight gain, amenorrhea, galactorrhea, diabetes
olanzapine (Zyprexa, Zydis)	constipation, dry mouth, weight gain, sedation, dizziness, akathisia, tremor, increased appetite, rhinitis, diabetes, hypercholesterolemia, elevated triglycerides, blurred vision, edema

Treatment

Table 4   **Adverse effects of medications used in the treatment of bipolar disorder (cont'd)**

Medication	Potential Adverse Effects*
quetiapine (Seroquel)	headache, dizziness, constipation, dry mouth, hypotension, sedation, rhinitis, diabetes, weight gain, hypercholesterolemia, elevated triglycerides, cataracts, arrhythmias
ziprasidone (Geodon)	nausea, constipation, diarrhea, dry mouth, sedation, dizziness, sialorrhea, headache, tremor, arrhythmias, weight gain
aripiprazole (Abilify)	headache, blurred vision, rhinitis, cough, tremor, anxiety, insomnia, nausea, sedation, constipation, sialorrhea, edema, weight gain

*Listed adverse effects are not exhaustive of side effects as reported in the Physicians' Desk Reference. More common effects were included, as well as some more serious effects. Any concern about an adverse effect from a medication should be discussed with your doctor.

†Does not have an FDA indication for bipolar disorder

when taken in the evening. In someone with poor appetite, a medication with associated increase in appetite may be desired.

Do not discontinue a medication when there is a suspected, bothersome side effect; speak with your doctor first. Some side effects are transient or can be easily alleviated by another remedy (e.g., ibuprofen for headache). Stopping medications abruptly when any side effect occurs may cause a **discontinuation syndrome**, as well as prematurely interrupt a potentially helpful treatment intervention. If possible it is best to remain on a medication for at least a few days, as some perceived side effects could be associated with unrelated conditions (e.g., viral infection). Bear in mind, scientific studies that compare an active medication to a placebo (sugar pill) have reported "side effects" in the placebo group as well. That said, if a suspected effect seems dangerous for any reason, it certainly is most

Discontinuation syndrome

physical and psychological symptoms that occur when a drug is suddenly stopped.

Table 5   Adverse effects of antidepressants by class

Medication class	Potential adverse effects*
SSRIs	nausea, diarrhea, insomnia, anxiety, nervousness, dizziness, somnolence, tremor, decreased libido, sweating, anorexia, dry mouth, headache, sexual dysfunction, serotonin syndrome
TCAs	dry mouth, constipation, nausea, anorexia, weight gain, sweating, increased appetite, nervousness, decreased libido, dizziness, tremor, somnolence, blurred vision, tachycardia, urinary hesitancy, hypotension, cardiac toxicity
MAOIs	dizziness, headache, drowsiness, hypotension, insomnia, agitation, dry mouth, constipation, nausea, urinary hesitancy, weight gain, edema, sexual dysfunction, increased liver enzymes, toxic food and drug interactions
Others (drugs listed separately)	
bupropion (Wellbutrin)	weight loss, dry mouth, rash, sweating, agitation, dizziness, insomnia, nausea, abdominal pain, weakness, headache, blurred vision, constipation, tremor, rapid heart rate, ringing in ears, seizures
venlafaxine (Effexor)	sweating, nausea, constipation, decreased appetite, vomiting, insomnia, somnolence, dry mouth, dizziness, nervousness, tremor, blurred vision, sexual dysfunction, rapid heart rate, hypertension
duloxetine (Cymbalta)	nausea, dry mouth, consitpation, loss of appetite, fatigue, drowsiness, dizziness, sweating, blurred vision, rash, itching, sexual dysfunction, tremor, unusual bleeding
mirtazapine (Remeron)	somnolence, appetite increase, weight gain, dizziness, dry mouth, constipation, hypotension, abnormal dreams, flu syndrome, low blood cell counts
nefazadone (Serzone)	somnolence, dry mouth, nausea, dizziness, insomnia, agitation, constipation, abnormal vision, confusion, liver failure
trazadone (Desyrel)	sedation, hypotension, dizziness, blurred vision, headache, loss of appetite, sweating, restlessness, rapid heart rate, prolonged erection

*Listed adverse effects are not exhaustive of side effects as reported in the Physicians' Desk Reference. Rather more common effects within each group were included, as well as some more serious effects. Side-effect profiles of medications within a class may vary. Any concern about an adverse effect from a medication should be discussed with your doctor.

Treatment

prudent to stop the medication until you are able to speak with your doctor, and if necessary be evaluated in an emergency setting.

43. Will I become addicted to the medication?

The one major concern for many patients who take psychotropic medications for years is the fear that they will become addicted to or dependent on their medication. **Addiction** is a complicated and controversial issue that bears some explaining. From a psychopathological or medical standpoint, addiction is defined as the pursuit of a substance in such a manner that the pursuit and use of it consumes so much time and energy for the person that he or she excludes the majority of, if not all, other important activities in his or her life. By that definition, anything that gives pleasure causing pursuit of it with abandon is potentially addictive—from gambling to sex to drugs to even the Internet and all variations on those themes. By that simple definition, no medication for the treatment of bipolar disorder other than the rare possibility of benzodiazepines, which are generally limited in use for that reason, has proven to be addictive.

Many people do, however, become physiologically dependent on various prescription medications, and this is where confusion reigns. Dependency has many definitions, which further confuses the picture. It is seen as a pejorative term, akin to addiction. But one confuses the concept of dependency as defined by the DSM-IV-TR with two other concepts, one being the dependency one has on any medication to treat a

Addiction

continued use of a mood-altering substance despite physical, psychological, or social harm. It is characterized by lack of control in the amount and frequency of use, cravings, continued use in the presence of adverse effects, denial of negative consequences, and tendency to abuse other mood-altering substances.

chronic illness that will flare up if the medication is stopped (e.g., diabetes, heart disease, or epilepsy as well as bipolar disorder); the other being that if one takes a medication chronically, then suddenly stops it and experiences withdrawal symptoms, he or she must be dependent on the medication. Dependency, instead, is more strictly defined in the DSM-IV-TR and is more akin to the previous description of addiction than the misunderstanding of the lay concept. There are two major criteria, the first being an emphasis on ever-increasing use in order to achieve a desired effect, known as tolerance; the second being that the concept of withdrawal includes both physiological and behavioral manifestations and is important in terms of the maintenance of the addictive behavior. This definition is very specific and as a result any physiological withdrawal symptoms that develop from the immediate cessation of a medication do not meet the definitional requirements of substance **dependence** unless they are accompanied by the other definitional criteria. This causes no end of confusion to both clinicians and the general public.

For example, the most obvious drug that people think about in terms of dependency includes most of the prescription pain medications that are called opiates (heroin is an opiate and was developed because it was thought to be nonaddictive). Everyone who takes these medications on a regular basis will develop some amount of withdrawal symptoms if they stop them abruptly. However, not everyone escalates their use of these medications over time, nor do they engage in reckless behavior in pursuit of the drug as the result of experiencing withdrawal symptoms. Because a drug

Treatment

Dependence
the body's reliance on a drug to function normally. Physical dependence results in withdrawal when the drug is stopped suddenly. Dependence should be contrasted with addiction.

like an opiate can make one high, is often pursued with abandon, and does cause dependency, people often mistake these two very different notions as one and the same.

Additionally, many medications that do not lead to addiction can cause physiological withdrawal. Many anticonvulsant medications, antihypertensive medications, and all steroid medications cause withdrawal, but no one would ever consider these drugs addictive. In stark contrast, many hallucinogens and stimulants do not cause any measurable physiologic changes in the body that one could absolutely label withdrawal, and nevertheless these are some of the most highly addictive substances known to humans. Where do antimanic agents, antidepressants, and other psychiatric medications fit on this continuum? Some antimanic agents are associated with various withdrawal syndromes, such as the possibility of a withdrawal **dyskinesia**, a transient movement disorder, associated with the abrupt withdrawal of a typical antipsychotic agent. Most antidepressants cause some level of physiologic dependency, especially the tricyclic antidepressants. Any drug, whether prescription medication or street drug, that causes a withdrawal syndrome must be tapered over time, or one risks developing withdrawal.

Dyskinesia

an impairment in the ability to control movements.

In fact, three types of discontinuation syndromes can occur when you stop a medication that you have been taking regularly for a significant period of time: withdrawal, rebound, and recurrence. Withdrawal occurs when a drug or medication is abruptly stopped. It is accompanied by clear physiologically measurable changes, including vital sign changes, skin color and temperature changes, and psychological distress. For some drugs, such as benzodiazepines, this can be a life-threatening emergency. For this reason, you must always consult a physician when deciding to discontinue a medication to see whether such a withdrawal could occur. Rebound occurs when the symptoms for which one was receiving the medication become transiently worse than the symptoms one had before treatment. This is a potential risk for any sleep medication from which rebound insomnia can be very severe. However, this is a transient effect and abates within days. Unfortunately, most people do not realize that rebound is expected and transient, and they immediately go back on their sleeping medications. Rebound generally is not accompanied by any physiologic changes. Recurrence is simply the return of symptoms for which one originally received the medication. Recurrence is more delayed in the timeline after stopping a medication than either withdrawal or rebound. Typically, if you begin to experience symptoms as early as a few days after stopping antidepressant medications, these actually represent rebound or minor withdrawal (no measurable physiologic changes) that is commonly known as a discontinuation syndrome. Rarely is it caused by recurrence. This is why it is a good idea to taper the medications. When the medications are appropriately tapered, any symptoms that return can properly be attributed to recurrence, and thus increasing the medication back to a therapeutic dose may be a wise choice. In summary, clearly, although many psychotropic medications can cause various discontinuation syndromes, they are *not* addictive.

Leslie's comments:

I know that I am not physically addicted to my medication, although I also know that if I were to go off of any of it I would have to do it slowly so that my brain chemistry could adjust to the changes. I do, however, know that I am dependent on the medication and it is frightening to think what might happen and how I would end up feeling if I didn't take it for a prolonged period of time. That fear makes me dependent but I also believe that being on the medication is like treating any other biologically-based illness: It is necessary to remain healthy.

44. Will I gain weight from the medication?

Weight gain is a very real concern for most patients. Unfortunately, the majority of medications used to treat bipolar disorder have some degree of weight gain associated with them. Both lithium and Depakote (valproate) are associated with weight gain, the mechanism of which is not understood. The weight gain from Depakote (valproate) may be associated with polycystic ovarian syndrome (see Question 79), but mostly it occurs independently of the condition. Weight gain from the anticonvulsants may not occur in everyone, so it need not immediately rule out a potentially effective treatment. It is important to maintain good nutrition and healthy eating habits, as well as partake in regular exercise, to help offset the weight gain risks. Being cognizant of any appetite-inducing effects of the medicine can help you resist urges to eat more as well. Of the atypical antipsychotics, Geodon (ziprasidone) and Abilify (aripiprazole) appear to have the least overall risk for weight gain, while Clozaril (clozapine) and Zyprexa (olanzapine) appear to have the highest risk. Aside from obesity, there is the associated risk of metabolic syndrome with atypical antipsychotics as well (Question 62). Anticonvulsants with lower risk for weight gain include Lamictal (lamotrigine) and Topamax (topiramate), although topiramate does not have FDA approval for bipolar disorder. Topamax (topiramate) has also been studied independently as a potential weight-loss agent and has been reported to reverse the weight gain caused by other agents.

In terms of the antidepressants, the older antidepressants have been classically associated with weight gain (tricyclics, monoamine oxidase inhibitors). When the SSRIs first entered the market, they were believed to have no associated weight gain as a group, and some even were found to cause weight loss (e.g., Sarafem [fluoxetine]). Keep in mind that side-effect profiles are typically developed from the early studies of medications, which are conducted over the short term (i.e., several weeks). In clinical practice, however, many physicians have found that SSRIs can be associated with weight gain over the long term. Although clinical trials have typically found that weight gain does not differ significantly from placebo, uncontrolled studies have noted weight gain over the long term. Paxil (paroxetine) appears to be more associated with weight gain clinically than the other SSRIs. Celexa (citalopram) has been reported to have early weight gain. There may be an increase in carbohydrate craving associated with SSRIs as a possible mechanism. Bupropion is one antidepressant that does not have weight gain associated with it and can be considered as one treatment option. More long-term controlled studies are needed to compare weight gain over time between antidepressant users and those who are not. Keeping in mind the potential for weight gain, good nutrition and exercise should be part of the treatment with antidepressants as well.

Ultimately, the risk for weight gain needs to be balanced against the risk for untreated bipolar disorder. Close monitoring of weight and vigilant efforts to prevent the initial weight gain can be very effective in limiting the amount that is gained. Weight gain on one agent does not necessitate the same on another agent, so different trials may be needed as well.

45. How long will I have to stay on medication?

It is important to understand that medications for bipolar disorder are used for treatment of the acute illness as well as to maintain **remission** of the illness. Remission may be partial or full, full remission occurring when there are no longer any symptoms. An acute manic episode is typically brought under control more quickly than an acute depressive episode. Full remission of symptoms, however, does not mean it is time to stop the medication. Many people stop their treatment prematurely because they either feel better or are experiencing side effects. It may be thought that the medication is not needed anymore or even questioned whether the medication had anything to do at all with the improvement (particularly if there were no side effects). Close monitoring by your doctor can help to address questions of efficacy as well as to provide the feedback as to level of improvement. When medication is discontinued prematurely, a relapse or recurrence is likely to occur soon thereafter. A relapse occurs if there is a return of symptoms of your previous episode within the period of time known as remission, which is within six months of resolution of symptoms. Recurrence occurs if the symptoms of either depression or mania return during the period of recovery, which is after six months of remission. Statistically

Remission

complete cessation of all symptoms associated with a specific mental illness. This occurs within the first six months of treatment, after which the term used is *recovery*.

speaking, after remission of either a manic or depressive episode, there is highest risk for recurrence within the first year. While the standard recommendation following one major depressive episode (unipolar) is to continue pharmacologic therapy for at least one year after remission, maintenance therapy will more likely be indefinite for bipolar disorder. The more episodes of either mania or depression you have over time increases the risk for future episodes. Bipolar disorder tends to worsen with time, particularly if left untreated, which is why indefinite treatment with a mood stabilizer is recommended. If an antidepressant is used, many clinicians recommend it be discontinued as soon as depressive symptoms have remitted, to reduce risk for a manic switch. Long-term management, however, will be guided by the frequency, severity, and consequences of past episodes.

46. Are both medication and therapy necessary in the treatment of bipolar disorder?

Both medication and therapy are necessary and effective treatments for both the depression and manic phases of bipolar disorder. In contrast to unipolar depression, therapy alone would not be adequate for the treatment of bipolar I disorder. And while medication is likely a necessary part of treatment for bipolar disorder, therapy too is usually a necessary adjunctive treatment to address the multitude of issues that can arise in treatment. Therapy can focus on potential precipitating stressors. In developing coping mechanisms and problem-solving abilities, the risk of recurrence under stressful circumstances in the future can be minimized. There may be situations when medication needs to be avoided during the depressed phase of the illness—the use of therapy, in particular cognitive-behavioral or interpersonal therapy, can sometimes make this possible.

The most important factor in determining a positive outcome from either modality is that both forms of treatment require *commitment* to the treatment in order for it to work. Therapy requires regular attendance to appointments; communication with the therapist during the session; and for some forms of therapy, work on assignments between sessions. The process of therapy is not easy. It can be anxiety provoking and one does not necessarily feel relief after each individual session. Relief comes over time with hard work on the issues. It may feel easier to cancel sessions or to terminate treatment prematurely, but then the therapy is not given a chance to be effective.

As for medication, its use requires daily compliance and regular communication with your doctor. It is often difficult for many people to remember to take a medication daily, twice a day, or more. Doses may be skipped. Missing doses regularly results in reduced efficacy of the medication. Sometimes a medication doesn't work right away. It becomes frustrating, and the medication treatment is abandoned prematurely. Often, when a person has a list of "ineffective" medications, many of them did not get adequate trials.

47. My doctor thinks I should have ECT. I thought that was no longer used. What is it and what does it do?

There are many myths surrounding the use of electro-convulsive therapy (ECT). ECT is a procedure that induces a seizure in the brain through an application of electric current through the scalp. ECT is not a first-line treatment (and is typically offered only after several failed medication trials or repeated hospitalizations), but it is a very effective treatment. It is very safe and is not painful. The patient is given anesthesia and a muscle relaxant for the procedure. For some patients, ECT is safer than medications, particularly for those with serious medical conditions for whom medication can be contraindicated, and for pregnant woman, who may not want to expose the fetus to certain medications (e.g., lithium). ECT is growing in use in elderly depressed patients because of higher rates of concurrent medical illness and risks of toxicity from medication. Psychotic depressions are often refractory to medication, and thus ECT may be considered early in the treatment to avoid a prolonged course of medication trials. ECT is an effective treatment for acute mania when it is unsafe to utilize medication.

The risk of serious complication from ECT is 1/1000. Cardiac complications are the most common adverse effects, which is why a pre-ECT evaluation includes evaluation of the cardiac system. Most potential cardiovascular complications can be avoided with the use of appropriate medications. Confusion and/or memory loss is also common. Confusion is usually transient. Memory deficits may be for events preceding or following the procedure. Memory deficits usually resolve over weeks to months after, although occasionally there are more persistent memory difficulties.

Although ECT provides rapid improvement in symptoms of depression and mania, there is a high rate of relapse—up to 50% within six months, so either continuation/maintenance ECT or medication is recommended following the treatment course. Continuation ECT is usually provided only if continuation medication has not successfully prevented relapse or recurrence of symptoms in the past.

ECT is usually done in a hospital setting as an inpatient (outpatient ECT may be provided for maintenance ECT). Medications are typically tapered off and discontinued prior to the treatment, and this process may need to occur in a hospital setting because of the risk for worsening depression and/or suicidality. ECT providers have received specialized training and certification. While protocols may vary from state to state, usually more than one physician needs to evaluate the patient and determine that ECT is clinically appropriate. Unfortunately, due to a negative portrayal of ECT by the media over the years, even with the safety features in place, this very effective procedure is highly stigmatized and even illegal in some jurisdictions.

48. Are there any natural remedies for bipolar disorder?

Alternative treatment

a treatment for a medical condition that has not undergone scientific studies to demonstrate its efficacy.

"Natural" or **alternative treatments** describe any treatment that has not been scientifically documented or identified as safe or effective for a certain medical condition. Examples of alternative treatments are acupuncture, yoga, herbal remedies, aromatherapy, biofeedback, and many others. In considering an alternative treatment, as with any scientifically documented treatment, you should consider the risks versus the benefits of such a treatment. If a particular procedure has no specific, direct risks associated with it, an important risk is potentially delayed treatment of the condition in question. For a mild depression, this risk may not be too great, but for a more severe depression with suicidal thoughts and certainly for an acute manic episode, it could be a fatal risk. Other risks include loss of money on an ineffective treatment, use of a treatment that is not standardized nor required to conform to specific regulations, and frustration when hopes of a unique treatment are not realized.

A number of dietary supplements have been touted to have effectiveness for depression, bipolar disorder, or mood lability in general, including St. John's wort, SAM-E, omega-3 fatty acids, folic acids and other B vitamins, magnesium, phenylalanine, and taurine. Although there is some promising, albeit early, evidence for efficacy or utility of some of these interventions, the evidence is too limited in scope to consider such treatments safe and/or effective.

Herbal remedies are a popular "natural" choice for treatment of many other conditions. A common assumption about these "natural" treatment choices is that they are safe because they are natural. While herbs are found in nature, as with manmade chemicals, herbs have a specific chemical structure that also alters the body chemistry. As such, there can be significant side effects from such compounds as well. Some of these side effects can be life threatening. For example, there have been many cases of liver failure from use of kava supplements around the world. In many cases, the problem per se is not that there are side effects, it is that the herbal treatments are not regulated as to either their safety or efficacy. If a specific treatment is known to be effective, there may be certain risks one is willing to take for relief. But without known efficacy it is not possible to make an informed decision as to the risks from exposure. Lack of regulation also means supplements available in the store are not rigorously tested for purity or quantity of the active compound in question. Individuals who sell these treatments may pose as experts but have not necessarily obtained any specialized training or certification. Keep these issues in mind if you choose to undertake an alternative treatment so that you can make fully informed decisions about treatment. Table 6 lists a number of popular herbal treatments and some of the problems that can arise if taking them while undergoing treatment for bipolar disorder.

49. Will diet or exercise help with my mood?

Bipolar disorder is not caused by problems with diet, although some believe that a balanced diet would leave one less predisposed to difficulties handling stress and thus possibly any mood conditions that result from that stress. Sleep, on the other hand, has a stronger association with bipolar disorder. During a manic episode, a person has a decreased need for sleep. Although poor sleep will not cause bipolar disorder, lack of sleep can precipitate a manic episode in a bipolar individual. Problems with sleep can predispose someone to depressive symptoms when chronically under-rested as well. Persons who sleep less then six hours per night have reduced concentration and irritability. In the management of bipolar disorder, development of good sleep hygiene is an important component of treatment for these reasons.

Table 6 Potential adverse effects and interactions of herbal substances in bipolar disorder

Herb	Adverse effects	Medication interactions
Ginseng	dizziness, heart palpitations, and an increase in heart rate, insomnia, mania, diarrhea, or allergic skin reactions	caffeine, hormone therapy, antipsychotics, insulin, diabetic therapy, or warfarin
Gingko Biloba	upset stomach, headaches, dizziness, heart palpitations, and allergic skin reactions	SSRIs, immunosuppressants, thiazide diuretics, warfarin, or NSAIDs
Ephedra / Ma Huang	increased heart rate, heart palpitations, difficulty urinating, dizziness, restlessness, insomnia, headache, low appetite, nausea, vomiting, tingling sensations and irritability; at high doses—increased blood pressure, irregular heart beat, heart failure, asphyxia, death	amitriptyline, dexamethasone, caffeine, theophylline, beta-blockers, urinary acidifiers or alkalinizers, diabetic therapy, and decongestants
St. John's Wort	stomach upset, fatigue, delayed hypersensitivity (allergic reactions), photosensitivity	birth control pills, antidepressants, narcotics, SSRIs, barbiturates, tetracycline
Kava Kava	stomach upset, headache, dizziness, drowsiness, liver failure	sedating medications, levodopa, barbiturates, alprazolam, and CNS depressants (including alcohol)
Melatonin	transient depression, headaches, general tiredness or drowsiness, abdominal cramps, irritability	CNS depressants, immunosuppressants

Treatment

Recent research has focused on the effects of exercise on mood and anxiety. Although the medical benefits of exercise are well known, the psychological benefits are less understood. Adults who exercise regularly report lower rates of depression and anxiety than the general population. Studies of the effect of exercise on depression have demonstrated positive results. Many theories exist as to how exercise improves mental health. Exercise causes changes in levels of serotonin, norepinephrine, and dopamine and causes the release of endorphins (which masks pain). It may reduce muscle tension, and adrenaline is released, which counteracts effects of stress. Psychologically too, exercise improves self-esteem, provides structure and routine, increases social contacts, and distracts from daily stress. Although the degree of impact that exercise has on mood disorders needs more research, there are many good reasons for including regular exercise as part of a treatment plan for bipolar disorder.

50. Why did my doctor recommend therapy if I am already taking medication?

Although therapy alone may be adequate for mild cases of depression, it is most optimal to be in therapy when taking medication for bipolar disorder. Studies on depression have shown that therapy and medication together have the best efficacy. Medication can treat your depression and mania independently of therapy, but it will not change environmental circumstances, will not change your coping skills, and will not change your personality or improve your self-esteem. Keeping in mind that depressive and manic episodes are typically due to a culmination of biological, psychological, and social factors, addressing the psychological and social underpinnings of your mood states is warranted. You cannot change your "biology" or genes, but you can use therapy to change other contributors to relapse. Ideally, the risk of future episodes can be reduced, as medication is generally not considered 100% effective in preventing recurrences of depression and mania. In fact, therapy may help minimize the use of antidepressant medication and thus reduce risk for switches into mania.

51. My mood stabilizer isn't helping. What happens next?

It can be disheartening when you do not feel better after a medication has been started. The reality is that the response rate to any given medication tends to be approximately 60% to 70% in clinical trials. This means that a good portion of individuals (more than 30%!) would not be expected to see improvement on the first medication tried. If a medication is not working, several factors first need to be considered: How long has the medicine been taken? Is the dose high enough? Is the medication being taken as prescribed?

Although antimanic medications for acute mania begin to work within days, it takes from four to six weeks (sometimes up to eight weeks) for the full effect of most psychotropic medications to work (after an adequate dose has been prescribed). Often the dose of medication has not been optimized. As long as there are few or tolerable side effects, the dose can be pushed to the maximum recommended dosage (Appendix B and C). Your doctor may want to go past the typical maximum dose on some medications (those that do not require blood tests to establish a therapeutic range) if you have no side effects and have partially responded to the treatment. In general, however, once the maximum dose has been prescribed for up to six weeks, and you have been taking it as prescribed, an adequate medication trial has occurred. If there is no improvement, your doctor should switch you to another medication. The change can even be within a class; for example, a lack of response to one antimanic agent does not mean the same will be true for another antimanic agent. If you have a partial response, your doctor may want to augment with another medication. **Augmentation** strategies generally involve using a medication with another mechanism of action so that different neurotransmitter systems can come into play to help, similar to what cardiologists do when they prescribe a second antihypertensive medication to patients whose blood pressure remains elevated after an initial antihypertensive has been prescribed. Thus, if treatment with a given agent fails, management techniques include switches within a class, switches to another class, augmentation, the use of medications other than those commonly prescribed, and finally ECT for more refractory episodes.

You must be open with your doctor about your level of adherence with a given medication. It is not unusual for people to forget doses or skip doses for specific reasons. People often do not want to admit this to their doctor, as they think he or she will become upset with them. If you are having problems with taking your medication, it is extremely important for your doctor to know so that the two of you can discuss some of the barriers to taking it, such as side effects. A lack of efficacy is often due to regularly missed doses, and without

Augmentation

in pharmacotherapy, a strategy of using a second medication to enhance the positive effects of an existing medication in the regimen.

this knowledge, other medication trials may be suggested unnecessarily.

52. Will the medication turn me into a zombie or make me look drugged up?

Looking "medicated" is often a reason some people shun treatment with various psychotropic medications. As a rule antidepressants do not typically cause such an effect. Medications that tend to be more sedating can make a person appear robotic or slow, but often these effects can be minimized or eliminated by changing the timing of the dosing or by switching to another agent. Traditional antipsychotic agents have a higher propensity for a certain type of side effect that can cause a robotic appearance. These medications are used less often in the treatment of bipolar disorder, but when they are utilized such side effects can be minimized with other types of medication. Some manic individuals feel as if they are overly slowed because they are used to and enjoy their highly energetic states when manic or hypomanic. In fact, their presentation usually appears more normal once the mania is under control. In the case of untreated depression, because of decreased energy, fatigue, and poor concentration, treatment is more likely to make you look less "robotic."

Some people worry their personality will be changed by medication. Medication does not change a personality. For someone who has been depressed for years (such as in **dysthymic** disorder) or hypomanic for years (such as in cyclothymia), it may seem as if the mood is just a part of his or her personality. Thus once your

Dysthymic

the presence of chronic, mild depressive symptoms.

depression or hypomania is treated, you might wonder if your personality has changed. Similarly, some people believe they will no longer experience sadness or joy and thus not feel human. Normal ups and downs, however, are not eliminated by antidepressant use.

Scott's comments:

I was afraid of this. Would I still be myself? A walking zombie? As I began my prescription, I felt no side effects. I was actually a bit leery of the efficacy of the medication, right up until the point that my wife said something to me that would have absolutely tripped my trigger in the past. This time, nothing happened. The physiological response was simply gone. Like water off a duck's back, her comment came and went, with no reaction from me. It was weird— normally I would have gone ballistic. This lack of sensitivity to stimuli that would have sent me into a manic state was simply amazing. Not having any other noticeable side effects was even more incredible. I look the same, I feel great.

Leslie's comments:

I was never afraid that the medication I was prescribed would turn me into a zombie, most likely because I had spent so much of my life being depressed that I welcomed any relief that I might get. I know that many people worry that taking medication will change their personality but again, I never had that fear. I quickly learned that medication allows my "real" personality to come out, rather than having the personality that is created as a result of the bipolar disorder; a personality that I believe is not my "real" self. I am concerned, however, when changes in my mood occur (for example, becoming depressed and sluggish) because I never know if it is a function of my medication, life's normal ups and downs, or the beginning of another bipolar episode.

53. My antidepressant is helping, but I have sexual side effects. What can I do?

Many antidepressants can have sexual side effects, which range from decreased interest in sex to difficulty having an orgasm. Many individuals are too embarrassed to ask their doctor about these problems, but it's important to discuss such side effects and learn your options. Depression itself can be a cause of reduced interest in sex, so first a determination needs to be made as to whether the depression has remitted on the medication. If depressive symptoms are gone, then other considerations should also be made, such as what the baseline sexual functioning was prior to becoming depressed or prior to the treatment. As a group, SSRIs do have a very high incidence of sexual side effects associated with them. These side effects can result in reduced compliance and thus reduced efficacy of the medication. Several options address these effects. Sometimes a "wait-and-see" approach is effective, as the negative effect may wane with time. Another option is to try another SSRI, which may not have the same effect for you personally, or to switch to a different class of antidepressant that does not typically cause sexual side effects. Antidepressants not typically associated with sexual side effects are bupropion, mirtazapine, and nefazodone. Nefazodone however, has been implicated in some cases of liver failure, and thus is not routinely prescribed unless other options have been exhausted. If the medication currently being taken is working, however, rather than take the risk of switching to another medication that may not be as effective, other types of medications may be prescribed in addition to the antidepressant that can counteract the effect SSRIs have on sexual functioning. The different options should be discussed with your doctor, but current approaches include the use of sildenafil (Viagra), bupropion, and herbal remedies.

54. I have episodes of hypomania without depressive episodes. I am considering not getting treatment.

Hypomanic symptoms by definition are not severe enough to cause marked distress or disability. To some degree, they may improve your general well-being and level of functioning. At the same time, however, such episodes can adversely impact your social relationships. Bipolar symptoms occur in cycles, and if you wait long enough, many symptoms may in fact remit even without treatment or you may cycle downward into a more depressive state. The real concern is whether or not someone will switch into a depressive state, which can be more debilitating. No one can predict with any degree of accuracy whether this will happen to you. Most studies of bipolar disorder have demonstrated that, on average, for every day one experiences hypomania, one will experience thirty-seven days of depression. The risks of a significant depression leading to disability are great: a loss of productivity in school or work, impaired relationships, family conflicts, financial problems, developmental delays in children, and most significantly, suicide. Research suggests that bipolar disorder itself can have harmful effects on the brain that render the cycles more frequent, intense, and prolonged with time. These effects may make you more susceptible to future depressive episodes, possibly more severe, in the future.

55. Can I take other medicines while I am on an antidepressant?

It is always important to inform any doctor you see of all medications you are taking, including any herbal or over-the-counter supplements. Although many medications can be taken concurrently, there is potential for reactions between many medications as well, thus consideration must be given for this. Sometimes, the potential reaction is minimal and may be due to additive side effects (e.g., sedating effects may combine). Other times, the presence of one medication can influence the elimination of the other medicine from the body, either allowing excessive accumulation or causing too-rapid depletion. Consequences can thus be toxicity or lack of efficacy. The SSRIs have specific enzyme groups that **metabolize** the medication. Each SSRI has a different profile as to the enzymes involved in its own metabolism. MAOIs are generally contraindicated in combination with all other antidepressants due to the risk for **serotonin syndrome**, which can be fatal (although there are certain combinations that skilled clinicians can prescribe in a methodical way to minimize the risks). Serotonin syndrome occurs when there is excess serotonin in the central nervous system. Symptoms include tremor, confusion, incoordination, sweating, shivering, and agitation. Most SSRIs are contraindicated in combination with thioridazine (Mellaril) as well, due to risk of **cardiac toxicity**. SSRIs should be used cautiously in combination with sibutramine (Imitrex), commonly prescribed for migraine,

Treatment

Metabolize

the process of breaking down a drug in the blood.

Serotonin syndrome

an extremely rare but life-threatening syndrome associated with the direct physiological effects of serotonin overload on the body. Symptoms include flushing, high fever, tachycardia, and seizures.

Cardiac toxicity

damage that occurs to the heart or coronary arteries as a result of medication side effects.

also due to risk for serotonin syndrome. St. John's wort, an herbal preparation used for depression, should be avoided when on a prescribed antidepressant, also due to potential risk for serotonin syndrome. Again, there are some circumstances when a psychiatrist will combine two SSRIs, for example, but this is typically done cautiously and under his or her guidance.

56. My internist is prescribing an antidepressant. How do I know if I should see a specialist? Should I see a psychiatrist?

A general practitioner of medicine can often adequately treat depression. There are situations, however, when a psychiatric consultation should be obtained. If comorbid conditions such as anxiety or substance abuse, severe suicidal thinking, or complicated personality issues exist, a psychiatrist is better equipped to manage the antidepressant treatment. In particular, the psychiatrist may be able to provide more frequent contacts and have longer sessions than the general practitioner typically has available. Two problems that arise when depression is treated by a general practitioner is the potential for under-dosing of medication as well as a too-short duration of treatment. Certainly if the depression is not responding to a prescribed treatment, consultation with a specialist is warranted as well. In the case of bipolar depression, however, or if there is concern because of a family history of bipolar disorder, it is usually best that a psychiatrist prescribe and monitor the symptoms, as management of the depression is typically more complicated.

Some individuals seek the services of a psychopharmacologist. The term can be somewhat misleading, as it implies a specialty in medication management of psychiatric conditions. In fact, all general psychiatrists are adequately trained in pharmacotherapy of mental disorders and need not be designated as psychopharmacologists. Some psychiatrists restrict their practice to medication management of mental disorders and thus are self-described as psychopharmacologists. There are psychiatrists who develop more expertise in the management of certain conditions and use of some medications, by virtue of clinical experience and perhaps research in academic settings, and thus may take referrals from other psychiatrists (and mental health clinicians) for more refractory conditions. In general, however, seeking consultation from a general psychiatrist is usually appropriate for most emotional problems. Specialists may be sought within the field of psychiatry for treatment of children and adolescents (child and adolescent psychiatrist), elderly (geriatric psychiatrist), medically ill (consultation-liaison psychiatrist), and individuals with substance abuse (addiction psychiatrists).

57. Why do I need a mood stabilizer with my antidepressant if I am depressed but not manic?

The term *mood stabilizer* has a variety of meanings attached to it. For the lay public, any medication that helps even out one's moods, including an antidepressant medication, is a mood stabilizer. For most psychiatrists the term *mood stabilizer* includes a class of medications that treat and prevent mania. These medications typically include anticonvulsant medications such as Depakote (valproic acid) and Equetro (carbamazepine); atypical antipsychotic medications such as Zyprexa (olanzapine), Seroquel (quetiapine), and Risperdal (risperidone); and lithium. The definition of a true mood stabilizer, however, is a medication that treats and prevents both depression and mania. There is no true mood stabilizer by that definition. Perhaps lithium comes the closest to meeting that definition, though it does not truly compare to antidepressants in effectively treating depression. Other antimanic medications that are never thought of as mood stabilizers include the anti-anxiety medications. At one time, alprazolam was used to treat certain forms of depression as well as anxiety and mania.

Thus, when a psychiatrist adds a "mood stabilizer" to an antidepressant you need to know exactly what class of agent is being prescribed and for what purpose. Many patients may have associated symptoms with their depression such as psychosis, and therefore an atypical antipsychotic medication is an appropriate addition to the antidepressant. Still other patients may experience a great deal of anxiety and panic, in which case the addition of an anti-anxiety agent may be appropriate. Some patients may never have had a manic episode, but some of their symptoms and family history are strongly suggestive of an underlying bipolar disorder. Under these circumstances, the safest medication to prescribe may be a mood stabilizer alone, unless the depression is severe enough to warrant aggressive care, in which case the psychiatrist may add an anticonvulsant, lithium, or an atypical antipsychotic as a preventative measure. Finally, some patients may only achieve a partial response to the antidepressant. When a partial response is achieved, the psychiatrist will typically add another medication to augment the primary medication's response rather than switch the medication altogether.

Leslie's comments:

I went to my primary care physician when I finally decided to get help with my illness. I was, unfortunately, misdiagnosed and as a result was treated only for depression. My physician prescribed an antidepressant, which caused me to become hypomanic and then plummet to the point of causing me to get into a car accident. My physician told me to stop taking the medication but I had terrible side effects as a result of that process. I then began seeing a psychiatrist, someone who specialized in the diagnosis and treatment of mental disorders. It was at that time that I was properly diagnosed with bipolar disorder and began my treatment with the medications that ultimately got my symptoms in check. That all happened about nine years ago and I now see a Clinical Nurse Specialist who is responsible for prescribing and monitoring my medication.

58. I have been prescribed a medication "off-label." Does that mean it is experimental?

The term *off-label* is used when a medication is used in a manner that is not FDA approved. Does this mean the medication is experimental? No, absolutely not. This means simply that no studies have been submitted to the FDA for approval of the medication for that particular use. It *does not mean* that no studies have been done. There are many studies that may not have been submitted, or that have been submitted and approved by European governments. It *does not mean* that the medication is not widely prescribed for a use other than what the FDA approved. It *does not mean* that doses under or over the recommended range approved by the FDA are neither effective nor safe. It *does not mean* that the medication is not safe in age groups younger or older than what the FDA approved. It merely means that when the company submitted the medication for approval to the FDA it submitted studies that specified a diagnosis, a dosage range, and an age group that their study subjects reflected.

Drug research and development have a fascinating history. Psychiatric drugs are often discovered serendipitously. Most drugs have multiple effects on the body, and focusing on one particular action to the exclusion of another is often as much a matter of marketing as it is drug action. For example, the first antipsychotic medication was developed and tested by a trauma surgeon who was specifically interested in finding a medication that could prevent surgical shock, a condition with a high mortality rate at the time. It was only through clinical observation that the medication was discovered to have antipsychotic effects as well as a variety of other effects on the body. The company that originally introduced it to the United States did not believe there would be a market for it as an antipsychotic and so released it to the public as an antiemetic. Only through multiple physician-driven lectures were psychiatrists in the United States comfortable enough to try it on patients suffering from schizophrenia. Perhaps even odder is the fact that the first antidepressant effects were observed in medications developed to treat tuberculosis. Only later was it discovered that these medications inhibited, or blocked, monoamine oxidase, an enzyme that breaks down norepinephrine, serotonin, and dopamine at the synaptic cleft.

To call any particular medication an antihypertensive, an antipsychotic, an antidepressant, or an anticonvulsant is actually a misnomer and really reflects the target population that a particular medication is geared toward when released to the public, not the broad range of effects of which the medication is capable. It also reflects the expense the companies go through in order to obtain FDA approval. The FDA requires that each medication target a specific diagnosis in order to receive approval, which is a hugely expensive enterprise for one diagnosis, much less for multiple diagnoses. Therefore, it is unlikely that drug companies will submit studies for approval for more than one or two diagnoses unless they can see some return on investment. As a result, clinical practice is often very different from what the PDR publishes. Clinical practice moves at a much faster pace than clinical trials and publications can keep up with. And while clinical trials are considered to be the definitive evidence of any particular medication's efficacy, astute clinical observations are what brought the biggest drug discoveries to the world and cannot be discounted simply because no study has yet to be published.

There are two broad reasons why off-label use makes sense in psychiatry. First, psychiatric diagnoses do not fit into the neat little categories the DSM-IV-TR attempts to define. They generally have many overlapping symptoms. For example, anhedonia, or loss of interest, can be seen in a number of conditions that include depression, schizophrenia, and frontal lobe damage. Many psychiatrists believe that medications should be prescribed to target the particular neurochemicals underlying such specific symptoms regardless of the DSM diagnosis. Off-label use is practiced with a clear rationale for another reason as well. Human nature defies categories. There may be broad similarities between two individuals suffering from depression, but it is doubtful that any one individual is suffering in exactly the same way as another from both a biochemical and psychological standpoint. Thus, one may respond to one particular therapy or antidepressant and not another, and the reasons are due to the therapies' and antidepressants' biochemical differences, not their similarities. For these reasons, off-label use in psychiatry is more the rule than the exception. Consider this example: a man sought out a cardiologist because he noticed getting palpitations from one particular brand of cola and not another. The cardiologist dismissed him outright. The man sought out another cardiologist who agreed to perform a stress test after he ingested the different brands, and sure enough, the man experienced premature ventricular beats with one particular brand of cola and not another. Never underestimate the power of one.

59. When is hospitalization necessary? What does it offer?

Hospitalization is the highest level of treatment. It is reserved for the most severe forms of mental illness. One criterion used for determining necessity of hospitalization is the presence of suicidality. Having suicidal ideation does not automatically dictate a hospital stay, but it does prompt an inquiry into the patient's level of risk to harm him or herself (or others). Hospitalization may also be indicated if a person's functional impairment is so poor that he or she is unable to adequately care for him- or herself (e.g., unable to get out of bed, not eating), such as in someone with severe depression. Most often, depressed individuals are willing to be hospitalized if recommended and thus do so voluntarily. There are situations, however, when the physician believes hospitalization is necessary but the patient refuses. This is more likely in cases of mania during which one rarely wants to be hospitalized. The physician then needs to decide if the person should be admitted involuntarily. Criteria for this process vary from state to state, but it is generally not easy to admit someone against his or her will. Most states have mental hygiene laws in place to protect patients' rights. Typically, dangerousness to self or others is the criterion required to commit someone. In that light, hospitalization for mania is usually due to potential for aggression, psychosis, or severe functional impairment that puts the individual at risk. Mental hygiene laws usually have an appeal process available for those committed involuntarily, and a reassessment is typically required within a specified time period as to necessity for continued hospitalization.

60. Can I drink wine with my mood stabilizer?

There are two parts to the answer to this question. The first part has to do with alcohol's effect on the brain of someone with bipolar disorder and the second part has to do with any drug–drug interactions between alcohol and your medication. First of all, alcohol is the last thing you want to put in your body if you suffer from bipolar disorder. Alcohol negatively affects the very chemicals that your mood-stabilizing medication is trying to normalize. Alcohol is a depressant. Alcohol is a euphoriant. Alcohol can worsen anxiety. Alcohol can worsen irritability. When alcohol is on board it acts as a sedative and can cause some areas of the brain to shut down their control of other more "primitive" areas of the brain, increasing impulsivity and reckless behavior. When alcohol washes out of your system your brain's activity level increases overall so that your moods end up cycling more rapidly and irritability and dysphoria can increase. Sleep is compromised as well, increasing your chances of relapsing into mania or depression.

In terms of any potential interactions between alcohol and bipolar medications, the answer is more complicated. With some medications like anticonvulsants and benzodiazepines the risk is serious insofar as there is a cumulative sedative effect of the two leading to an increased probability of intoxication and possible respiratory suppression. With other medications, such as the atypical antipsychotics, the risk of having a seizure, while small, is increased. With certain antidepressant medications, such as the monoamine oxidase inhibitors, the risk is serious, as the interaction with some forms of alcohol, particularly red wines, can lead to **malignant hypertension**, which is potentially life threatening. With tricyclic antidepressants, the risks are again due to their sedative effects, which are additive to alcohol, and thus cause intoxication and its incumbent risks more readily. Finally, with the newer SSRIs, the additive effects are much less noticeable, as these medications are not found to be sedating nor to affect cognition and motor coordination adversely. Given both the potential for worsening illness, as well as exacerbating symptoms, it is best to avoid alcohol altogether.

Malignant hypertension

elevated blood pressure that is acute and rapidly progressive with severe symptoms, including headache.

Scott's comments:

The first time I had alcohol while on medication was on my wedding anniversary. My wife and I were staying at a beautiful resort, and decided we'd celebrate with a glass of wine at dinner. That night I had the most incredibly violent dreams that I've ever had. My sleep was interrupted with horrible nightmares about bloodshed and killing. The next morning I discussed this with my wife—it was enough to make me swear off alcohol.

61. Are there long-term dangers to taking medication?

With the recent press regarding the link between Vioxx and heart disease, and the alleged link between antidepressant medications and suicide, fear of long-term adverse effects has grown, particularly for newer medications. With respect to psychiatric medications, this fear includes the belief that medication is a form of mind control that can have permanent long-term effects on one's personality and mind. This particular idea is categorically false. No medication has that level of control over one's mind. With respect to potential long-term adverse effects of various bipolar agents, however, one should be aware of each agent's particular issues. The most common and/or concerning issue for each is the subject of the following paragraphs. The list is otherwise too long; refer to the package insert for each drug for a complete list.

Lithium

Lithium is the most well known in terms of potential adverse effects. First, it is important to note that blood

Therapeutic index

the ratio between the toxic dose and the therapeutic dose of a drug, used as a measure of the relative safety of the drug for a particular treatment.

Hypothyroidism

decreased or absence of thyroid hormone, which is secreted by an endocrine gland near the throat and has wide metabolic effects. When thyroid hormone is low, metabolism can slow, leading to symptoms that can mimic clinical depression.

levels need to be monitored regularly. Lithium has a very narrow **therapeutic index**—that is, the blood level for minimum effectiveness and the blood level for potential toxicity is fairly narrow. Second, there are three potentially long-term adverse effects of which to be aware and to understand: **hypothyroidism**, kidney damage, and weight gain. There are a number of risk factors for developing hypothyroidism. They include having a prior history of thyroid problems, being female, being overweight, having a family history of thyroid problems, having rapid-cycling bipolar disorder, and requiring higher doses of lithium. When hypothyroidism develops as a result of lithium it is generally reversible, unless antibodies to thyroid are present. The best indicator for presence of antibodies is family history. If hypothyroidism occurs, thyroid replacement may be indicated. The most common problem that occurs to the kidney in response to lithium is the inability to concentrate urine and preserve fluid over time. The risk of this is both dose and time dependent. That is, kidney toxicity generally occurs after taking higher doses of lithium for many (ten to fifteen) years. Chronic renal failure can occur at this time; lithium needs to be discontinued once this has happened. One should avoid taking nonsteroidal anti-inflammatory medications for extended periods of time as these medications increase the blood level of lithium and can also adversely impact the kidneys. Weight gain associated with lithium is a slow onset effect. It occurs for a variety of reasons, including the initial increased thirst associated with lithium, the possibility of hypothyroidism from lithium (which can also cause weight gain), and the effect of lithium itself on metabolism. Risk factors associated with weight gain include being young, overweight, and female. The odds of gaining weight are about 50/50.

Depakote (valproate)

Depakote (valproate) has some immediate and long-term adverse effects. The immediate concern for various blood disorders prompts monitoring of a complete blood count. **Thrombocytopenia**, a drop in platelets (important in blood clotting), is a not uncommon effect. This is easily reversible by stopping the medication. **Hepatitis** and **pancreatitis** can also occur early on in treatment, and for this reason liver function tests should be performed regularly. Women of childbearing age should be cautioned, as Depakote (valproate) is associated with a higher incidence of birth defects. A more common, less dangerous, but more distressing problem is alopecia, or hair loss. This is also reversible with discontinuation of the medication. Weight gain is a potential problem, and Depakote (valproate) may play a role in the development of polycystic ovarian syndrome (Question 79).

Equetro (carbamazepine)

Although reported infrequently, serious adverse organ system effects have been observed with the use of Equetro (carbamazepine). Early in treatment a rash is possible. Most rashes are benign. Should signs and symptoms of a severe skin reaction such as **Stevens-Johnson syndrome** appear, Equetro (carbamazepine) should be withdrawn immediately. Blood cell problems are the most well known complications. Both **leucopenia** (loss of white blood cells) and thrombocytopenia can occur. In addition, the liver can be adversely affected, resulting in hepatitis and jaundice. Equetro (carbamazepine) levels, a complete blood count, and liver function must be monitored throughout treatment in order to detect as early as possible signs and symptoms of a possible blood or liver problem. Equetro

Treatment

Thrombocytopenia
an abnormal decrease in the number of platelets in the blood.

Hepatitis
inflammation of the liver, caused by infection or a toxin.

Pancreatitis
inflammation of the pancreas.

Stevens-Johnson syndrome
a severe inflammatory eruption of the skin and mucous membranes that can occur as an allergic reaction to a medication.

Leucopenia
an abnormal lowering of the white blood cell count.

137

(carbamazepine) should be discontinued if any evidence of a significant problem appears. Long-term toxicity studies in rats have indicated a potential carcinogenic risk; however, no evidence exists that this medication is carcinogenic in humans. In women of childbearing potential, Equetro (carbamazepine) should be avoided whenever possible or prescribed as monotherapy because the incidence of congenital abnormalities in the offspring of women treated with more than one anticonvulsant is greater (see Question 80).

Atypical Antipsychotic Medications

Although the FDA treats the atypical antipsychotics as a class in terms of side effect profiles, all coming with the same warnings on their package inserts, they do not all demonstrate the same adverse effects equally. The most concerning class effect is the development of metabolic syndrome, which is characterized by a number of metabolic changes, including weight gain and elevated cholesterol, triglycerides, and fasting blood sugars. Some patients have gone on to develop diabetes. A few have developed diabetic ketoacidosis, a medical emergency stemming from extremely high blood sugars. Not all of the atypical antipsychotics appear to cause this problem to the same degree. The two worst offenders are Clozaril (clozapine) and Zyprexa (olanzapine). This is unfortunate, because Clozaril (clozapine) is the most effective antipsychotic on the market, and many clinicians swear by Zyprexa (olanzapine) as being the second most effective and perhaps best-tolerated agent. In the middle are Risperdal (risperidone) and Seroquel (quetiapine). Geodon (ziprasidone) and Abilify (aripiprazole) appear to have no effect on the development of metabolic syndrome though both have been known to cause weight gain to a lesser degree than the others. All of these medications have been known to lead to cerebrovascular events in the elderly, and so their use in this population should be minimized. They also appear to increase the rate of mortality from all conditions in this population for unknown reasons. Finally, while the development of **extrapyramidal** side effects and **tardive dyskinesia** is greatly reduced in this class compared to the older typical antipsychotics, it is not nonexistent. Again, it appears some are more likely than others to cause extrapyramidal problems, particularly Risperdal (risperidone). Risperdal (risperidone) also can elevate prolactin, which has a number of adverse consequences, including breast growth, lactation, and decreased libido.

Selective Serotonin Reuptake Inhibitors (SSRIs)

SSRIs have been on the market since the introduction of Prozac in the late 1980s. Numerous studies have attempted to link them to long-term dangers such as cancer or other medical conditions aside from their psychological effects. None of these studies has yet held up to any scrutiny. All of the studies linking SSRIs to suicidal behavior analyze data at the beginning of treatment and most likely represent an unidentified side effect that can be associated with suicidal behavior. Such side effects could be increasing anxiety and insomnia or an extrapyramidal side effect that causes patients to become uncomfortably restless (**akathisia**). Another factor that may be involved is the improvement in energy levels that often occurs before an improvement in mood, which may result in increased motivation and energy to act on suicidal desires. This is why close monitoring during the initial phase of treatment with these medications is imperative.

Extrapyramidal

the parts of the brain responsible for static motor control. The basal ganglia are part of this system. Deficits in this system result in involuntary movement disorders. Antipsychotic medications affect these areas, leading to extrapyramidal side effects, which include muscle spasms (dystonias), tremors (Parkinson's), shuffling gait, restlessness (akathisia), and tardive dyskinesias.

Tardive dyskinesia

a late-onset involuntary movement disorder, often irreversible, typically of the mouth, tongue, or lips, and less commonly of the limbs and trunk. These movements are a consequence of long-term antipsychotic use but are less commonly observed with the newer, atypical antipsychotics.

Akathisia

a subjective sense of inner restlessness resulting in the need to keep moving. Objectively, restless movements or pacing may be signs of akathisia.

Treatment

139

62. What is metabolic syndrome and how does it relate to mood stabilizers?

If you have three or more of the following you are diagnosed with metabolic syndrome:

- A waistline of 40 inches or more for men and 35 inches or more for women (measured across the belly)
- A blood pressure of 130/85 mm Hg or higher
- A triglyceride level above 150 mg/dl
- A fasting blood glucose (sugar) level greater than 100 mg/dl
- A high-density lipoprotein level (HDL) less than 40 mg/dl (men) or less than 50 mg/dl (women)

This syndrome is important to mental health for the following reasons. Metabolic syndrome, more often than not, is caused by obesity. Bipolar disorder may increase the risk of obesity and metabolic syndrome due to changes in energy related to mood variability. The severity and chronicity of bipolar disorder may also affect the incidence of obesity. The number of previous episodes is positively correlated with being overweight or obese. The greatest gain in weight for bipolar patients is during the acute phase of their treatment. Obese individuals tend to have a more severe and intractable type of illness. There is some preliminary evidence that treating severe obesity may improve mood, at least depression. At Danbury Hospital in Connecticut, the bariatric surgery department has been following its patients for several years now and documenting the changes in medication as a result of weight loss. They have found that with the reduction in weight, and the resulting reduction in fasting blood sugars, triglycerides, and cholesterol, a significant number of the patients eventually no longer require antidepressant medication. It is not clear if the same effect occurs with bipolar patients, as there are just too few of these patients in the program to have any reliable numbers.

Finally, the medications used to stabilize mood may cause weight gain and/or metabolic syndrome. It appears that just about all the medications used to treat bipolar disorder, old and new, lead to weight gain. Of the atypical antipsychotics, the medications that cause the most weight gain, in order of most significant to almost negligible, include Clozaril (clozapine), Zyprexa (olanzapine), Risperdal (risperidone), Seroquel (quetiapine), Geodon (ziprasidone), and Abilify (aripiprazole). These medications have also been implicated in elevated fasting blood sugars, elevated cholesterol and triglycerides, and rarely the development of diabetes (again in descending order). Although these two risks are related, it is possible to develop any one of them without the others. The traditional mood stabilizers lithium and Depakote (valproate) can also cause weight gain, but have not been shown to cause metabolic syndrome. In fact, some evidence suggests that adding Depakote (valproate) to Risperdal (risperidone) lowers the cholesterol in Risperdal (risperidone) users. These weight changes are most dramatic in thinner individuals. But being overweight prior to treatment conveys its own risks, particularly the risks of precipitating or worsening metabolic syndrome. You should work with both your internist and psychiatrist to choose medications that are most effective with the fewest side effects.

Strategies you can take to reduce the chances of weight gain during treatment include changing your diet, increasing exercise, and/or choosing medications less associated with weight gain. These include mood stabilizers such as Trileptal (oxcarbamazepine) or Lamictal (lamotrigine), or the lowest-risk atypical antipsychotics such as Geodon (ziprasidone) or Abilify (aripiprazole). In addition, a combination of medications can be taken that can either reverse or reduce the risk of weight gain. These combinations include a variety of off-label strategies such as adding Topamax (topiramate), Symmetrel (amantadine), metformin, or Pepcid to Zyprexa (olanzapine). All of these strategies carry a degree of risk, and to date none have proven to be universally effective.

63. Why did my doctor prescribe an antipsychotic for me when I am just depressed?

Antipsychotic medications are often prescribed for patients suffering from psychotic symptoms resulting from their depression. Such symptoms often revolve around false beliefs that the patient deserves some horrible punishment for a minor transgression the patient believes to be a major sin or crime. Antipsychotics specifically target those symptoms, thus relieving patients of those painful thoughts and feelings. With the introduction of newer antipsychotic medications, however, their use as augmenting agents to antidepressants even in the absence of psychosis has become a new option for psychiatrists.

The newer antipsychotic medications, called atypical antipsychotics or second-generation antipsychotics (SGAs), were developed because of increasing concern regarding the risk of developing a severe, potentially irreversible movement disorder known as tardive dyskinesia. Patients suffering from mood disorders are at greater risk for developing this movement disorder than patients who suffer primarily from psychotic disorders. SGAs have reduced this risk dramatically. They are, as a result, generally safer to use than their predecessors, although recently there have been growing concerns about their metabolic effects on the body, including the potential for weight gain, increased blood sugar, and increased cholesterol and lipids. Despite these concerns, they remain an effective strategy when patients are showing only a partial response to their antidepressant medication or have a history of bipolar disorder and need medication to prevent the possibility of mania while undergoing treatment with an antidepressant medication.

64. How does generic medication differ from trade names?

The generic name of a medication is the international scientific name for the molecule that constitutes the active form of the medication. The company that develops the medication applies for a patent and obtains exclusive rights to sell the medication. They then give the medication a trade name. This trade name can change from country to country and from its intended use. For example, the medication with the generic name paroxetine is marketed under the trade name Paxil in the United States and Seroxat in the United Kingdom. The medication with the generic name bupropion is used as an antidepressant under the trade name Wellbutrin and as a smoking cessation medication under the name Zyban. The medication with the generic name fluoxetine is used under the trade name Prozac as an antidepressant and as

Sarafem, a medication prescribed by obstetricians, for women suffering from premenstrual symptoms. Once a medication goes off patent, other companies obtain the right to make it and sell it. At this point generic forms of the medication that may be less expensive become available. These medications are sold under their generic names. As physicians first know the original form of the medication by its trade name, the physicians often continue to write prescriptions under that name. By law pharmacies must fill the prescription with the less-expensive form of the medication unless the physician specifically indicates to the pharmacy not to substitute. As a result the filled prescription will come back to the patient under the generic name rather than the trade name.

Are there differences between generic medications and medications under the trade name? The active ingredients of the medication are identical. The "fillers" or inactive ingredients making up the rest of the medication may differ. There may also be more percentage variations between the amounts of active ingredients from pill to pill in generic medications than in trade medications as the requirements for quantity control are more stringent with trade medications than with generic medications. Generic medications can vary by ±20% in bioavailability (the amount of medication that reaches the bloodstream). Different companies can manufacture generics so each time you get a refill on a generic you may get a different one with different bioavailability. For many medications, these differences are so minute as to be negligible, and with repeated dosing the differences cancel each other out. However, some drugs used to treat bipolar disorder, such as Depakote, Depakote

ER, Eskalith, Lithobid, and Equetro have a narrow therapeutic index (NTI). With NTI drugs, small variances in the blood levels may cause changes in the effectiveness or toxicity of that drug. Many insurance plans will cover both the brand name drugs and the generics, although some drugs have no generic substitution. Physicians may indicate "dispense as written" to ensure a brand name drug is dispensed by the pharmacist.

65. Are mood stabilizers prescribed for reasons other than bipolar disorder?

The term *mood stabilizer* typically refers to a medication with antimanic properties and is actually a misnomer (see Questions 41 and 58). Most psychoactive medications have multiple effects and the decision to label a particular medication a mood stabilizer, an antidepressant, an anticonvulsant, an antipsychotic, or an anxiolytic is often as much a matter of marketing as it is due to the drug's clinical effects. The newer class of psychotropic medications known as atypical antipsychotic medications, for example, were developed and designed as antischizophrenic medications. Only later were they tested and marketed as mood stabilizers. Because of their relatively benign safety profile compared with their earlier counterparts (Haldol (haloperidol) and chlorpromazine, for example), however, they have been used as both antianxiety medications and sedative/hypnotic medications. More recently they are being studied for use in both unipolar and bipolar depression.

Thus, mood stabilizers have multiple properties that are utilized by different physicians to target specific symptoms with which their patients present. For example, neurologists have long been using mood stabilizers that are anticonvulsants to treat epilepsy, but also to prevent migraine headaches and other pain syndromes. Many patients with panic disorder who do not respond to SSRIs (e.g., Sarafem [fluoxetine]) will respond to the anticonvulsant medication valproic acid. But mood stabilizers have been used in the treatment of other anxiety disorders, including generalized anxiety disorder, obsessive-compulsive disorder, and posttraumatic stress disorder. The atypical antipsychotics have been found to be especially useful in severe obsessive-compulsive disorder in which the obsessions are intractable. Seroquel (quetiapine) has been found to be especially useful in managing insomnia associated with drug and alcohol dependency and psychosis in patients suffering from Parkinson's disease, and it has been used as an alternative to the benzodiazepines in managing anxiety. See Table 7 for a list of conditions that mood stabilizers can treat.

Table 7

Conditions for which mood stabilizers are utilized
Mood disorders
Anxiety disorders
Impulse control disorders
Sleep disorders
Seizure disorders
Migraines

PART V

Associated Conditions

I have been diagnosed with bipolar disorder and anxiety. How is the combination of conditions treated?

My spouse is drinking a lot of alcohol lately. My friend thinks he might be self-medicating. What does that mean?

Why is my doctor telling me I need treatment for my addiction when I thought treating the depression would solve my problem?

More ...

66. I have been diagnosed with bipolar disorder and anxiety. How is the combination of conditions treated?

Anxiety is a condition that commonly occurs with bipolar disorder, particularly in the manic phase of the illness, but can also occur in the depressive phase or co-occur as an independent condition. The easiest way to think about this is that if you only have anxiety in the manic or depressive phase of the illness and it abates when your mood stabilizes, then it is a symptom of the bipolar disorder and not an independent condition. The type of anxiety associated with mania is on a level far more extreme than generalized anxiety. People commonly describe it as a restless energy that will not allow them to sit still. It is often accompanied by irritability and racing or disorganized thoughts. Sometimes the anxiety results because your ambitious grandiose schemes are being thwarted by others who cannot understand the vast rewards completion of such schemes will bring.

Some anxiety conditions, such as social phobia, panic disorder, and generalized anxiety disorder, can cycle with your moods, essentially abating during the hypomanic or manic phase but returning during euthymia and even worsening during the depressive phase. The treatment for anxiety in the context of bipolar disorder is tricky. The SSRIs are a very useful treatment for many anxiety disorders but are less than ideal in persons who suffer from both anxiety and bipolar disorder. The benzodiazepines, which can be very beneficial in aborting panic attacks, are also tricky because the rate of alcoholism and drug abuse is high among bipolar individuals.

The first task in treatment is to control the bipolar disorder as best as possible. Fortunately, many of the anticonvulsant agents affect GABA, the major neurotransmitter implicated in many anxiety disorders, and therefore they can have anxiolytic and antipanic effects independent of their mood-stabilizing properties. If the anxiety abates with mood stabilization you are in luck. If not, the problem is a bit trickier. Some anxiety conditions, such as posttraumatic stress disorder and obsessive-compulsive disorder, respond preferentially to SSRIs, and SSRIs are clearly trickier to use in bipolar disorder, as mentioned previously. If the symptoms are generally in check, cognitive-behavioral therapy is the treatment of choice. If an SSRI is warranted, remaining on an antimanic agent is imperative prior to its initiation. A combination of therapy and medication is typically the best treatment approach for a variety of anxiety disorders, such as generalized anxiety disorder, panic disorder, social anxiety disorder, and obsessive-compulsive disorder.

Scott's comments:

This was my diagnosis exactly. My anxiety is being treated with Klonopin, which I find highly effective. Combined with my bipolar medication, I feel like normal now. The behaviors that I used to exhibit are no longer part of my persona, but memories of days past. The thought of trying to tough it out with both bipolar disorder and anxiety disorder just seems way too hard when modern medicine is available to treat these conditions so specifically. Better living through chemistry, indeed.

67. My spouse is drinking a lot of alcohol lately. My friend thinks he might be self-medicating. What does that mean?

Individuals with a mood disorder may abuse alcohol or drugs in a misguided effort to feel better. In the case of depression, alcohol can initially give the impression of improving one's mood, but in actuality, alcohol is a depressant. Likewise, use of drugs to get "high" is usually followed by a "crash" during which the mood becomes sad or despondent. During mania, both poor impulse control and recklessness can result in alcohol and/or drug abuse. Such substances, however, serve to further exacerbate the condition and can contribute to a crash into depression. Depression can sometimes be caused by the alcohol or drug abuse itself and will remit when abstinence is achieved. Often depression precedes the alcohol or drug use, and people turn to these substances in an effort to feel better. Typically though, feeling better really just means being "numb" or deadened to the depressed feelings. Treatment of the depression and/or mania may result in achievement of abstinence. This of course will depend on the stage of substance abuse. If the individual has become dependent on (addicted to) the alcohol or drugs, then concordant substance abuse treatment will likely be necessary as well. As long as the person is addicted to alcohol or drugs, recovery from bipolar disorder will be limited. In fact, substance abuse is a problem that needs to be considered if someone is refractory to treatments for bipolar disorder. Seeing a person who specializes in treatment of addictions would also be helpful as there are different forms of therapeutic interventions often needed in persons who have addiction. In addition, there are specialized treatment programs for persons with both bipolar disorder and substance abuse.

68. Why is my doctor telling me I need treatment for my addiction when I thought treating the depression would solve my problem?

Patients with a combination of addiction and depression are at higher risk for suicide, homicide, poor compliance, relapse, and greater hospitalization rates. Although there is some evidence to support the concept that many patients use substances to "self-medicate" an underlying depression, there is no evidence that antidepressant medication leads to abstinence. Although the "self-medication hypothesis" may seem right for some individuals, once an addiction develops it takes on a life of its own. It is unlikely that medicating it away can conquer addiction. Also, if you continue to use drugs or alcohol while receiving antidepressant medication, they render antidepressant medication essentially ineffective. Thus depression can not be effectively treated without also treating the addiction. However linked they may have been in their origins, they are now separate entities that both require treatment in order for you to return to health.

69. How are alcoholism and bipolar disorder connected?

Bipolar disorder and alcoholism do co-occur at higher-than-expected rates. No one knows why but it appears, surprisingly, that they are not genetically linked. Bipolar men who are alcoholics often had a family history of alcoholism when compared with nonalcoholic bipolar men. Alcoholism among bipolar women, however, was not associated with a family history of alcoholism. Instead, their addiction often stemmed from anxiety and depression. Bipolar women have a higher risk of developing alcoholism than non-bipolar women. The rate in bipolar women for alcoholism is 29%, and in bipolar men it is 49%.

More importantly, alcohol, cocaine, heroin, PCP, and marijuana can all cause mood swings that make everyone using these drugs suspect of having a mood disorder in general and bipolar disorder more specifically. When these patients are hospitalized psychiatrically as a result of an impulsive, potentially dangerous behavior in the context of their drug and alcohol abuse, the likelihood of their being discharged on a "cocktail" of psychiatric medications with a diagnosis of bipolar disorder is high. With average lengths of stay in a psychiatric hospital of about a week the accuracy of such a diagnosis is suspect at best. The proof is not even in the pudding, because complicating the picture is the fact that the medications one is discharged on are symptom and not diagnostic specific. Therefore, although one's mood may stabilize with an anticonvulsant agent or antipsychotic, that does not mean one has bipolar disorder. Unfortunately, the pitfall inherent in the diagnosis is that all too often these patients and their families focus entirely on the bipolar diagnosis, attributing continued relapse into drugs and alcohol to bipolar disorder while doing nothing to get treatment for substance or alcohol abuse. But, as was discussed in Question 60, alcohol and drugs of abuse worsen bipolar symptoms and go further toward explaining the mood swings than vice versa. More likely, any mood swings stand a far better chance of improvement from abstinence than from any psychotropic medication offered.

70. Are individuals with bipolar disorder at risk for drug abuse?

Alcohol and drug abuse is very common among people with bipolar disorder. The most common co-occurring illnesses with bipolar disorder are substance abuse disorders, with up to 60% of patients with bipolar disorder having substance-related problems. Substance abuse can make bipolar disorder more severe and worsen the course of the disease by exacerbating symptoms or precipitating episodes. Such comorbidity may result from the self-medication of mood disorder symptoms, or mood symptoms may be induced by substance abuse. The risk of comorbid substance abuse may be increased by family history of substance use, an early age of onset of bipolar disorder, and the presence of mixed episodes. Treatment for co-occurring substance abuse, when present, is an important part of the overall treatment plan. The diagnosis of bipolar disorder should not be made in the presence of active substance use, as many illicit drugs (and the rapid withdrawal from them) can cause symptoms of mania (and subsequent depression). Ideally the substance of use is discontinued so that a baseline of functioning can be assessed. Symptoms should dissipate if due to an ingested substance. If substance abuse persists, treatment for presumed bipolar disorder may be initiated if co-occurring substance abuse treatment is obtained. Even if self-medication of symptoms was the reason illicit substance use was initiated, once abuse or dependence has set in, the problem will require separate treatment.

71. Since returning from active duty overseas, my husband is having rageful episodes, is irritable, is suspicious of others and complains of racing thoughts at night. Is he bipolar?

Active duty can be a precipitating stressor for many mental disorders. As part of any evaluation, various diagnoses are considered because of overlapping symptoms. A common combat casualty for many soldiers returning from war is posttraumatic stress disorder (PTSD). Symptoms of PTSD can look very much like a mood disorder, and in fact untreated PTSD often results in development of depression and substance abuse. In some studies as many as 52% of subjects develop alcohol abuse or dependence and 47% develop depression. In a person who is at higher risk for bipolar disorder, it is certainly plausible that the first episode would occur following as stressful an event as active duty in combat. In fact, in a recent NIMH-funded study, a high percentage of persons diagnosed with bipolar disorder also exhibited symptoms of PTSD. Symptoms of PTSD may look like bipolar disorder, however. PTSD is associated with three primary symptoms that persist for longer than a month after a traumatic event:

- **Re-experiencing**, such as flashbacks or nightmares or intense memories
- **Hyperarousal**, such as jumping at noises one used to ignore
- **Numbing**, such as an inability to feel pleasure and a tendency to isolate

With re-experiencing, there are recurrent, intrusive thoughts and images in the mind. The patient may

Re-experiencing

the phenomenon of having a previous lived experience vividly recalled and accompanied by the same strong emotions one originally experienced.

Hyperarousal

a heightened state of alertness to external and internal stimuli, often resulting in sleep disturbance, problems concentrating, hypervigilance, and exaggerated startle response. Typically seen in post-traumatic conditions.

Numbing

the psychological process of becoming resistant to external stimuli so that previously pleasurable activities become less desirable.

exhibit behavior as if the event were recurring, and intense psychological distress can occur. Re-experiencing can result in irritability and agitation. Racing thoughts may actually be the recurrent memories and **ruminations**. Symptoms of hyperarousal include difficulty sleeping, outbursts of anger, difficulty concentrating, and hypervigilance. Symptoms of numbing include detachment and avoidance, which can look like depression. The cluster of symptoms can thus look very much like bipolar disorder. In a recent study of U.S. soldiers returning from Iraq, about 16% said they were experiencing symptoms of depression and anxiety. Although their symptoms are likely to be caused by PTSD, it is important to rule out bipolar disorder because the treatment for PTSD is typically an antidepressant, which would not be indicated during an acute hypomanic or manic episode. The sad truth is, though, that many if not most soldiers will not admit to having a problem or seek help. They have been trained to "suck it up," and they consider any admission of emotional problems related to their duty as an admission of weakness in the face of their responsibility. The earlier your spouse gets into treatment, the better the chance for a positive outcome.

Ruminations
obsessive thinking over an idea or decision.

72. What are the similarities and differences between borderline personality disorder and bipolar disorder?

The distinction between bipolar disorder and borderline personality disorder is one of the most hotly studied and debated issues today in terms of research and clinical care. The greatest debate occurs regarding the bipolar spectrum disorders, although bipolar I disorder shares some elements with borderline personality disorder as well. The two extreme arguments range from negating bipolar II/bipolar NOS disorders that overlap with borderline personality disorder to negating borderline personality disorder, with the arguments from most clinicians and researchers falling somewhere in between. Although bipolar II is a relatively new disorder and was not operationalized until the publication of DSM-IV in 1994, this debate has been ongoing since the criteria for borderline personality disorder were first established in 1980 with the publication of DSM-III. Borderline personality disorder is characterized by a pervasive pattern of instability of interpersonal relationships, self-image, and **affects,** as well as marked impulsivity. Symptoms begin by early adulthood and include:

Affect

feeling or emotion, especially as manifested by facial expression or body language.

- Frantic efforts to avoid real or imagined abandonment
- Extremes of idealization and devaluation of interpersonal relationships
- Markedly and persistent unstable self-image or sense of self
- **Impulsivity** in at least two areas that are potentially self-damaging (e.g., spending, sex, substance abuse, reckless driving, binge eating)
- **Recurrent suicidal behavior**, gestures or threats, or self-mutilating behavior
- **Affective instability** due to a marked reactivity of mood (e.g., intense episodic dysphoria, irritability, or anxiety)
- Chronic feelings of emptiness
- **Inappropriate, intense anger or difficulty controlling anger** (e.g., frequent displays of temper, constant anger, recurrent physical fights)

- Transient, stress-related paranoia or severe dissociative symptoms

The symptoms noted in bold are similar to those that occur during a hypomanic or manic episode, which is where the overlap in diagnosis can occur. The other criteria, however, are more distinct and characterize or are associated with the long-standing troubled interpersonal relationships.

The history of the term *borderline personality* is an interesting one. Originally the term was used to describe patients whose symptoms traversed the border between "neurosis" and psychosis. The individuals were considered "pseudoneurotic schizophrenics" because their general ability to adapt was profoundly impaired although superficially they appeared unremarkable. Borderline patients can in fact become transiently psychotic in the midst of one of their rages, but later such patients were characterized instead as having emotionally unstable personalities. In 1975 the psychiatrist Otto Kernberg conceptualized borderline personality disorder as a diagnosis associated with particular primitive **defense mechanisms**, of which **splitting** was one. The criterion regarding patients' tendency to overidealize or devalue another person is an example of splitting, in which they have difficulty integrating the good and bad in people and thus "split" the person into either all good or all bad. Personality traits are thought to be different from symptoms associated with mood disorders in that they are a reflection of enduring patterns of perceiving, relating to, and thinking about the environment relative to oneself and are exhibited in a wide range of contexts. These traits

Associated Conditions

Defense mechanisms

a set of unconscious methods to protect one's personality from unpleasant thoughts and realities that may cause anxiety.

Splitting

a defense mechanism that serves to separate opposing affective or emotional states, such as in overidealizing a person one day and devaluing the same person the next. The ability for the ego to hold more than one representation of an object is impaired.

are generally first recognized in adolescence and endure throughout adult life.

A recent study examining the affective instability common to both borderline personality and bipolar II disorder patients found clear differences between the types of affects associated with the two disorders. Borderline personality disorder was associated with greater mood lability in terms of anger, anxiety, and depression/anxiety oscillation, while bipolar II disorder was associated with greater mood lability in terms of depression, elation, and depression/elation oscillation. In fact, the study also showed that labile anger alone was sufficient to predict (with 72% accuracy) the diagnosis of borderline personality disorder versus another personality disorder. This finding is surprising, given the fact that bipolar II disorder is considered to be more often associated with irritability than bipolar I disorder, which is more associated with euphoria or elation. Additionally, another clear distinction exists in the underlying sense of self between the two disorders. Patients with borderline personality disorder suffer from feelings of emptiness with strong fears of abandonment—feelings that are always present even when the mood is generally stable. Bipolar patients, on the other hand, have a generally stable sense of self when their moods are stabilized.

Leaving aside the validity of such a reconceptualization of the two diagnostic categories, whether or not there is utility to this approach is the more important question. After all, the ultimate goal of establishing diagnostic accuracy is for the purposes of treatment. With the newer antipsychotic medications that are now approved for bipolar disorder, the utilization of pharmacological interventions for treating a condition that was once thought to be solely amenable to long-term psychotherapy offers new hope for these patients. Keep in mind, however, that such medications are neither diagnostic nor symptom specific and therefore a positive response does not ensure diagnostic validity. Increasing research in this area has demonstrated some modest success in stabilization of borderline personality symptoms with combinations of mood stabilizers and/or antipsychotics. The emphasis on psychotherapy, however, continues to be the primary mode of treatment for patients with borderline personality disorder. The most utilized and validated psychotherapeutic technique for borderline personality disorder is dialectical behavior therapy, designed and studied by Dr. Marsha Linehan. This technique focuses on behaviors and less so on feelings except with respect to how they link directly to self-injury. Studies in Europe have demonstrated a decrease in both suicidal and self-destructive behaviors, though effect on mood is less certain.

73. Is there an overlap between ADHD and bipolar disorder?

Attention-deficit hyperactivity disorder (ADHD) is a condition distinct from bipolar disorder, but the differentiation of mania from ADHD can be difficult. There are similarities in symptoms, particularly in the differential diagnosis of children and adolescents. It has been argued that ADHD is misdiagnosed in some young people who actually have bipolar disorder, although a high number of youth with bipolar disorder also have ADHD. The coexistence of the two conditions may be related to the age of onset of bipolar disorder, as adults with a reported history of comorbid

Associated Conditions

ADHD tend to have the onset of bipolar disorder before age 19. Studies of rates of ADHD in the children of bipolar adults have found higher rates than in control subjects.

Both disorders share many characteristics such as impulsivity, inattention, hyperactivity, high physical energy, mood swings, frequent coexistence of conduct disorder and oppositional-defiant disorder, and learning problems. Family history in both conditions often has the presence of mood disorders. Elevated mood and grandiosity are the symptoms best able to distinguish between pediatric bipolar disorder and ADHD. Also, with bipolar disorder, hyperactivity may be more episodic. Irritability, hyperactivity, accelerated speech, and distractibility are frequent in both childhood-onset bipolar disorder and ADHD and are not useful in differentiating between the two disorders. The response or lack of response to stimulant medications is not diagnostically helpful, but classification of the diagnosis is important as stimulants can promote mania in a bipolar individual if not on a mood stabilizer first (as with antidepressants).

PART VI

Special Populations

Do children get bipolar disorder?

How is childhood bipolar disorder different
from adult bipolar disorder?

What are the risks for suicide in children
and adolescents?

More . . .

74. Do children get bipolar disorder?

Bipolar disorder was once thought to occur only rarely in youth, with the peak age of onset in the early thirties. However, approximately 20% of all bipolar patients have their first episode during adolescence, with a peak age of onset between 15 and 19 years of age. Rates of bipolar disorder in children, once considered extremely low, are now thought to be closer to rates in adults, although due to questions of diagnostic reliability, true rates are not known. It is known that 20% to 30% of youth with major depression go on to develop bipolar disorder. The DSM-IV-TR criteria for bipolar disorder are not believed to adequately describe the symptoms present in childhood, which is why the disorder is often missed in the younger age groups. Depression as well was once believed to be rare in children, but symptoms of major depression are now known to occur. Rates of mood disorders in general in children have been rising over the past half-century for unclear reasons. Bipolar illness in childhood is more likely to affect the offspring of parents with bipolar disorder. While manic symptoms are the same in children as described for adults, the duration criteria are believed to be too long for diagnosis in children. The mood shifts between mania, depression, and euthymia can occur several times within a day. In addition, children with mania are more likely to be irritable than elated. Older bipolar adolescents are more likely to have presentations similar to adults. In children, it may be difficult to distinguish bipolar disorder from attention-deficit hyperactivity disorder, oppositional-defiant disorder, conduct disorder, developmental disorders, or anxiety disorders. Although there remains debate and controversy over the diagnosis of mania in children, it is increasingly recognized that there are children with severe affective dysregulation manifested by severe tantrums, destructiveness, and aggression that may in fact be early bipolar disorder. In fact, childhood onset mania is often considered more chronic rather than episodic, most likely with a mixed (with depression) presentation and psychotic features more common. Early-onset substance abuse may signal bipolar disorder as well.

75. How is childhood bipolar disorder different from adult bipolar disorder?

Childhood bipolar disorder is not given specific diagnostic criteria in the DSM-IV-TR because the criteria for bipolar disorder are considered applicable to all age groups. The younger the age of onset, however, the less the disorder looks as described in the DSM. Prepubertal-onset bipolar disorder tends to be a nonspecific, chronic, rapid-cycling mixed manic state. For adolescent onset, the presentation of mania is more closely matched to the adult presentation. It is more likely, however, that depression precedes mania in an adolescent. The onset of bipolar disorder in patients with a history of ADHD is often between 11 and 12 years of age. Many children who develop bipolar disorder develop a depressive disorder first. Of youth with major depression, up to a third go on to develop mania/bipolar disorder.

Studies have shown that observation of five behavioral symptoms in children/early adolescents aid in correctly diagnosing childhood bipolar disorder. Manic symptoms that do not overlap with ADHD are elation, grandiosity, flight of ideas/racing thoughts, a decreased need for sleep, and hypersexuality (in the absence of sexual abuse or overstimulation). As opposed to adults, however, children with mania seldom experience euphoric mood; the most common mood disturbance is severe irritability with "affective storms" (prolonged and aggressive temper outbursts). In between outbursts, these children are described as persistently irritable or angry. Manic children do often have a decreased need for sleep—they can function well on less sleep than normal. Due to their aggressiveness, these children frequently receive a diagnosis of conduct disorder. Aggressive symptoms often result in the psychiatric hospitalization of manic children.

76. What are the risks for suicide in children and adolescents?

Suicide is a very real risk for depressed youth. Suicide is the third leading cause of death in teenagers. One in five people with bipolar disorder commits suicide. A study by the Centers for Disease Control and Prevention of high school students indicated that nearly 20% of teens had seriously considered suicide and that more than 1 in 12 had made a suicide attempt in the previous year. Male teens are more likely to kill themselves, while more females attempt suicide. The majority of teen suicides are with guns. Children also can have suicidal ideation but are less apt to make attempts the younger they are. Risk factors for suicide include:

- Previous suicide attempts
- Depression
- Alcohol or substance abuse
- Family history of psychiatric illness
- Stressful circumstances
- Access to guns
- Exposure to other teens who have committed suicide

Stressful life events tend to be higher in children and adolescents who attempt suicide and may include loss of family members due to death or separation, physical or sexual abuse, frequent arguing in the home, or witnessing violence. Youth who are grappling with their sexual identity are particularly at high risk for suicide. Suicidal youth tend to have poor social adjustment and are lacking adequate social supports. Bipolar youth are at increased risk due to higher rates of mixed mania and depression along with poor impulse control.

Some depressed adolescents engage in self-injurious behavior of cutting themselves without the specific intention of killing themselves, a symptom that is more typical in persons who experience a chronic emptiness and "emotional numbness." The pain from cutting is described as a relief because the physical pain detracts from the emotional pain. Such behaviors are a sign that help is needed and is typically seen in depression when occurring in adolescence, but it is also a feature in some personality disorders in adults. While those who engage in self-injurious behaviors don't necessarily intend to kill themselves, "accidental death" is a risk as well as the development of permanent scarring. Often the cutting behavior is transient, occurring during particularly stressful periods (e.g., loss of relationship) and dissipates with the development of better coping skills and improved impulse control.

77. What is the treatment approach for children and adolescents?

The treatment of children and adolescents must first begin with a comprehensive evaluation by a qualified practitioner. Find a treatment provider who has experience with this population or better yet has specialty training with this population. The evaluation tends to encompass more areas of query than do adult evaluations, with full developmental history and family history obtained, and school functioning assessed and contrasted with home functioning. As in adults, other conditions must be considered and ruled out before diagnosing a mood disorder. Once bipolar disorder has been diagnosed, a treatment plan should address the following needs:

- Individual
- Medical
- Family
- School
- Legal

Individual needs can be addressed with psychotherapy. Cognitive-behavioral and interpersonal therapy approaches have been studied and found effective in adolescent depression. Children and adolescents can benefit from other psychotherapeutic approaches as well. Group therapy should be considered if there are concerns about social development. In addition to individual psychotherapy, work with children and adolescents often needs some level of family work, either with the parents or including siblings as well. Because a child is a member of a family system, the dynamics between the child and others may need to be addressed in ways that individual work cannot. Problems with behavior may require enhancement of parenting skills. Psychoeducation of family members too may be needed to help them understand the patient's illness.

Medically, a decision is to be made regarding the use of **somatic** treatments for bipolar disorder in a child or

Somatic

referring to the body. Somatic therapy refers to all treatments that have direct physiological effects, such as medication and ECT. Somatic complaints refer to all physical complaints that refer to the body, such as aches and pains.

adolescent, such as a mood stabilizer. Due to the severity of untreated bipolar disorder, a medication will likely be recommended in addition to therapy. All children and adolescents should have medical clearance through the pediatrician to rule out any underlying medical conditions. Baseline laboratory studies will be needed.

Educational needs are also assessed in children and adolescents. A child with bipolar disorder needs and is entitled to accommodations in school. Bipolar disorder and the medications used to treat it can affect a child's school attendance, alertness and concentration, motivation, and energy available for learning. Functioning can vary greatly at different times throughout the school year. Recurrence of depressive and manic episodes can cause academic delays and may be associated with comorbid learning disabilities. A board of education assessment will determine the most appropriate educational setting. The educational needs of a particular child with bipolar disorder vary depending on the frequency, severity, and duration of episodes of illness. Most states mandate that appropriate educational services be made available to minors with emotional and/or behavioral problems, which may consist of smaller classroom settings, non-public school placement, day treatment programs, or even residential treatment settings.

Legal needs of a child also have to be considered in the evaluation process. As the child is a minor, a parent or guardian will make the final decision regarding the treatment intervention. Older adolescents do, however, have some say about their treatment. In particular, it is best if they are in agreement to a medication because they cannot be forced to take a medication against their will. Other legal issues to consider are custody issues and need for family court involvement or state involvement.

78. What are the risks of treating my teenager with psychotropic medication?

In years past, it was often presumed that medications worked in young people the same as in adults. Clinical trials rarely included persons under the age of 18. Prior to the development of SSRIs, children and adolescents were rarely treated with antidepressants. The tricyclics and monoamine oxidase inhibitors that were available had potentially harmful side effect profiles that out-weighed the benefit of the treatment. This was in part because clinical studies in persons under 18 did not demonstrate antidepressants to be more effective than placebo. When SSRIs entered the market, however, because of their better safety profile, prescriptions for antidepressants in children and adolescents increased dramatically. There was clearly a need for safe, effective treatments, because in adults untreated depression has serious adverse outcomes. In recent years, studies of SSRIs have been conducted in children and adolescent populations, with efficacy demonstrated in some. One observation from SSRI studies (that was also noted in the early studies using tricyclics) was the presence of a relatively high placebo response rate. Adolescents may benefit from the supportive contact with the treatment provider and thus "respond" to the placebo. Talk ther-apy is clearly a necessary part of treating depression in children and adolescents, even if on medication.

In the treatment of bipolar disorder, medication use is more complicated due to the potential need for more than one medication. In addition, except for the use of Sarafem (fluoxetine) for major depression, no medication indicated for a mood disorder (depression or bipolar) in adults has such an indication for use in children or adolescents. Some antidepressants, for example, while effective in adults have data that do not support their efficacy in children and adolescents. Although the FDA has not provided indications for use of medications in youth with bipolar disorder, because of the significant risks of no medication intervention, it is standard practice to treat the condition with medications that have demonstrated efficacy in adults. Many medications have some level of research evidence in literature supporting their use in childhood bipolar disorder, but their use is considered "off-label." Monitoring of medication therapy must be done very closely.

In the case of using various mood stabilizers other than antidepressants, choices become more difficult due to the increased severity of side effects in contrast to SSRI antidepressants. Children and adolescents appear to be more sensitive to the side effect of weight gain, for example, which can significantly hamper compliance as well as contribute to physical health problems. Lithium has been studied in children for a variety of conditions. Adverse effects are similar as in adults, with careful monitoring of kidney and thyroid function required. Regular blood level monitoring is necessary as well because of the narrow range between effective blood level and toxic blood level. Studies in patients with epilepsy have shown that Depakote (valproate) may increase testosterone levels in teenage girls and produce polycystic ovary syndrome in women who begin taking the medication before age 20 (Question 79). Therefore, young female patients taking Depakote (valproate) should be monitored carefully by a physician.

There have been recent concerns about the risk for increased suicidal thinking in children and adolescents prescribed SSRIs. Warnings are now included in the labeling of all antidepressants that there can be a risk of suicidality, and close monitoring is recommended. It is not clear, however, if such effects are specific to certain SSRIs. A recent analysis by the FDA of all the studies of newer antidepressants showed a rate of suicidal behaviors in 3% to 4% of children and adolescents with depression who took an antidepressant and a rate of 1% to 2% of those taking a placebo (inactive pill). Of note, there were no deaths by suicide in any of the studies. Also, there was no difference in the rate of suicidal behavior for those being treated with an antidepressant for an anxiety disorder. The results of the analysis have prompted the FDA to require a warning on all antidepressants regarding the risk of increased suicidal behavior (thoughts or actions) when used in children and adolescents. While this can be disconcerting for any parent, it is important to keep in mind that the risk for suicide in untreated depression is approximately 15%. Reasons for the increased rate while on medication may be due to some of the factors described in Question 61, but it is not understood at this time. The necessity for close monitoring is important because of this. As in adults, depression is a condition that is associated with suicidality. Whether on an antidepressant or not, patients need to be closely monitored for the onset of such symptoms or worsening of existing symptoms. Keeping the data in mind, contrary to fears of increased suicidal tendencies, data from around the world actually document that the suicide rate among teenagers has dropped concordant with increased prescribing of SSRIs for depression.

79. I have been hearing about polycystic ovaries. What is that and should I be concerned if I take Depakote (valproate)?

Polycystic ovary syndrome, also known as PCOS, is a syndrome that includes a cluster of signs and symptoms usually associated with having polycystic ovaries. A polycystic ovary is defined by having at least ten ovarian cysts. Not all women with polycystic ovaries develop PCOS and not all women with PCOS have polycystic ovaries. The signs and symptoms may include polycystic ovaries, menstrual cycle irregularities (both frequency and flow), excessive body and facial hair (hirsutism), female-patterned baldness, and skin problems, including acne. All of these signs and symptoms stem from hormonal imbalances, which include an overproduction of testosterone. Additionally, truncal obesity and metabolic syndrome may accompany the signs and symptoms described above.

The prevalence of PCOS varies depending upon the researchers' definition but ranges anywhere from 4% to 18%. PCOS does appear to occur more often in women with epilepsy than others, with rates between 13% and 25%. It also appears to occur more frequently in women with bipolar disorder, though in frequencies less than in those with epilepsy. Menstrual irregularities have been shown to approach 50% in women with bipolar disorder independent of treatment. One explanation as to why women with either epilepsy or bipolar disorder may have more frequent menstrual irregularities, as well as PCOS, may have to do with the brain's poor regulation of the endocrine system secondary to seizures or manic-depressive cycles (see Question 27). Not only is it believed that these conditions may cause PCOS, it may be the case that PCOS worsens these conditions through the hormonal imbalance PCOS causes. The question of whether or not PCOS is caused by anticonvulsant medications, especially valproic acid, has been hotly debated, though current research suggests that valproic acid does increase the chance of developing it. This research has suffered from the fact that few, if any, longitudinal studies following women over a long course of therapy have been done. That being said, the increased risk is particularly evident in young teenage women. The mechanism by which Depakote (valproate) may increase risk is poorly understood but may be attributed to a number of factors. Depakote (valproate) appears to affect hormone levels independently, which may in turn contribute to PCOS. Depakote (valproate) is not enzyme inducing and therefore will not reduce hormones that promote PCOS as other anticonvulsants will do, such as Equetro (carbamazepine), phenytoin, and Lamictal (lamotrigine). In fact, the latter two anticonvulsants appear to reverse PCOS in women who develop it while on Depakote (valproate). Finally, Depakote (valproate) causes weight gain, which is associated with higher circulating levels of insulin and male hormones, both being linked to PCOS. It is difficult to determine diagnostically whether or not one has PCOS as there are different definitions of the syndrome and no one test can clinch the diagnosis. As a result it remains a diagnosis of exclusion. The simplest approach in management of PCOS is to treat the symptoms empirically. That is, if there is a strong possibility it is developing or has developed, switching medication is the first line of treatment.

80. I want to get pregnant but take medication for bipolar disorder. What can I do?

Because bipolar disorder has its average onset in late adolescence and early adulthood, many women with bipolar disorder are faced with decisions about their treatment in the midst of their reproductive years. The best first step is to plan the steps to take *before* becoming pregnant. You need to familiarize yourself with the data that are available regarding medication use and its potential effect on a fetus. You also need to be aware of the risks associated with stopping medication treatment. First off, know that there is controversy in the literature as to whether or not bipolar disorder improves during pregnancy, but that even if it does for some, it does not for others. Also, it is important to know that there is a high risk for symptom recurrence in the immediate postpartum period.

The risk of use of mood-stabilizing agents during pregnancy appears to be greatest in the first trimester, although there are **teratogenic** effects that can occur later as well. A review of the literature on various medications was done by Yonkers et al. (Am J Psychiatry 161:4, April 2004) and noted the following:

Teratogenic

that which can interfere with normal embryonic development.

Lithium

There is an association with cardiovascular malformations. Ebstein's anomaly occurs in 0.1% to 0.2% of the offspring of lithium users in contrast to 0.005% in the general population. While the risk is increased several-fold, the absolute risk remains small. Lithium-exposed infants have been found to weigh more than nonexposed infants. In two studies of behavior and development, there were no differences in milestone development or behavior. Exposure to lithium during labor has been associated with "floppy baby syndrome," so close monitoring of levels is part of routine obstetrical care.

Depakote (valproate)

Use during the first trimester is associated with high rates of neural tube defects of 5% to 9% with the risk being dose related. Craniofacial abnormalities, growth retardation, small head circumference, and heart defects are at a twofold increased risk from the use of anticonvulsants. Depakote (valproate) has neonatal complications associated with it as well such as heart rate decelerations, irritability, jitteriness, feeding problems, and abnormal tone. Some experts recommend Depakote (valproate) be switched to another mood stabilizer before pregnancy. Teratogenic risk is also higher with the use of more than one anticonvulsant agent.

Equetro (carbamazepine)

Craniofacial defects, fingernail hypoplasia, and developmental delay have been found at high rates. Neural tube defects range between 0.5% and 1%. Reduced birth weight and head circumference are associated with Equetro (carbamazepine) use. Equetro (carbamazepine) is not recommended by most experts for use during pregnancy unless there are no other options.

Lamictal (lamotrigine)

In 2004, rates of major malformations appeared to be similar to those in the general population, but new information suggests an increased risk for cleft lip and palate with first trimester exposure.

Typical Antipsychotics

There have been mixed findings on whether there is an increased rate of malformations, with many studies conducted on chlorpromazine. One study on rates between those on chlorpromazine for psychosis and those who were psychotic but not on chlorpromazine showed similar rates of malformations that were higher than in the general population, suggesting that something else about the illness was contributory. Case reports have suggested a link between Haldol (haloperidol) and limb reductions, but larger case series have not supported this. The risk from typical antipsychotics is considered by many experts to be less than the risk from some mood stabilizers, and thus during pregnancy, a switch from a mood stabilizer to an antipsychotic is often made.

Atypical Antipsychotics

There are limited data on the use of atypical antipsychotics in pregnancy.

Keeping the data in mind, it is possible to manage both pregnancy and bipolar disorder safely, but again the planning should ideally occur before getting pregnant. With careful planning and monitoring, outcomes can be improved for both mother and offspring. Communication with both psychiatrist and obstetrician are critical.

81. I found out I am three months pregnant and have been on a mood stabilizer. Is my baby at risk?

Question 80 goes over the findings in the literature on the use of various medications for bipolar illness during pregnancy. Although it is ideal that planning for conception occur first, for many women pregnancy is not anticipated. Unfortunately, many of the fetal malformations do occur in the first days to weeks after conception and thus by the time pregnancy is discovered, the exposure has often already occurred. Depending upon the medication being taken, once that time period of higher risk has passed, it may no longer be prudent to go off a specific medication. Keep in mind as well that although rates are higher than the general population for various malformations, in some cases the rates with medication exposure are still low. Meetings with both your psychiatrist and obstetrician to go over your options are needed as soon as possible. Prenatal testing for some conditions may be desired to check for abnormalities. Your psychiatrist can work with you to minimize additional risk for the duration of the pregnancy and to determine the best course of treatment postpartum.

82. Can I take a mood stabilizer or antidepressant while I am nursing?

Data regarding use of many medications during breastfeeding are scarce. The FDA gives a category classification for most medications as to whether they are safe during pregnancy or nursing, but this information is not always reliably based upon available data. Some medications, like benzodiazepines, are known to be present in large quantities in breast milk and thus are presumed to be unsafe. There have been increasing amounts of data as well as interest in the risks versus the benefits of taking bipolar medications while breastfeeding. Typical medications taken for bipolar disorder may include both antidepressants and mood stabilizers, such as anticonvulsants and/or antipsychotics.

All antidepressants are excreted into breast milk. Although differences may exist between antidepressants as to quantities found in breast milk, data are insufficient to make definitive statements about these differences. Both tricyclic antidepressants (TCAs) and SSRIs are generally undetectable in nursing infant blood. Nortriptyline has been the most studied TCA in breastfeeding women. Children exposed to TCAs have been followed through preschool, and no developmental differences have been found compared to children not exposed to TCAs. TCAs, however, are not typically the first-line treatment for depression because of their side effects and are not recommended in bipolar depression. Data are available on the use of Sarafem (fluoxetine), Zoloft (sertraline), Paxil (paroxetine), Celexa (citalopram), and Luvox (fluvoxamine), with Zoloft (sertraline) being studied most over the past few years. Although SSRI medications have not usually been detectable in most studies, there have been infrequent reports of detectable serum levels of Zoloft (sertraline), Celexa (citalopram), and Sarafem (fluoxetine) in exposed infants. A case report on paroxetine found no evidence of it in breast milk, thought possibly due to its **half-life**, but more studies are needed. No adverse developmental or behavioral effects have been detected to date in nursing infants, but there have been no long-term studies. Zoloft (sertraline) is generally considered relatively low-risk, but Sarafem (fluoxetine) may have some level of risk associated with it, possibly due to its long half-life. Three cases of colic have been reported in babies with detectable levels of Sarafem (fluoxetine), and there is some evidence for reduced weight gain after birth. Although for the most part levels of SSRIs are not usually detectable in infant serum, this does not exclude the possibility of the drug having entered the central nervous system. In unipolar depression, the benefits of breastfeeding may outweigh the risks of

Half-life

the time it takes for half of the blood concentration of a medication to be eliminated from the body. Half-life determines as well the time to equilibrium of a drug in the blood and determines the frequency of dosing to achieve that equilibrium.

SSRI exposure alone, and thus staying on medication while nursing is often warranted.

In considering use of other medications for bipolar disorder while nursing, data too are limited. Lithium levels in breast milk are close to half the levels in maternal blood. Infant kidney function is not optimal, which can result in elevated blood levels of lithium. If lithium is taken during breastfeeding, the infant's blood levels and complete blood count should be monitored closely. Depakote (valproate) has not been associated with adverse effects in exposed infants or mothers, and the American Academy of Neurology does advocate breastfeeding for mothers on antiseizure medication. Equetro (carbamazepine) levels in breast milk are low. The American Academy of Pediatrics lists both Depakote (valproate) and Equetro (carbamazepine) as compatible with breastfeeding. As for the antipsychotic agents, there had been twenty-eight reports on infant exposure during breastfeeding at the time of the Yonkers et al. review (see Question 80); no adverse events were reported in the majority of cases.

Deciding whether to breastfeed while on bipolar medications is difficult. The risk of going off medication, however, is great. There is a high rate of recurrence of illness during the postpartum period. Lithium has been found to reduce the rate of relapse from 50% to less than 10% in the postpartum period. Although it is desirous of many women to breastfeed, if you absolutely do not want the infant exposed to any medications, the more conservative approach is to remain on medication and not breastfeed, as both depression and mania can be associated with adverse outcomes in an infant. Untreated maternal depression is associated with reduced weight gain in infants. A depressed or manic mother will be less in tune with a baby's needs, less able to monitor the environment for safety, and less apt to engage in a nonverbal dialogue with the baby. Early **attachment** is important in a baby's development, as poor attachment early on confers risks later in life for emotional and behavioral problems.

83. Are there any medications I should avoid if I have bipolar disorder?

The medications you should be concerned about can be divided into two broad categories—those that may *directly* provoke or exacerbate mania and those that interact negatively with medications used to treat bipolar disorder. In addition to prescription medication, there are over-the-counter medications, street drugs, and herbal remedies that should be avoided and are thus being lumped into the category of "medications" here. Medications that provoke or exacerbate mania can be divided into four subcategories:

- Antidepressants and stimulants used commonly to treat psychiatric and neurological conditions
- Steroids and beta agonists used commonly to treat pulmonary conditions
- Dopamine agonists used commonly to treat neurological conditions
- Over-the-counter medications and street drugs that are stimulants and hallucinogens

Antidepressants cause the most concern among patients and clinicians alike for two main reasons: they may cause switching to mania and/or they may cause mood to destabilize, leading to worsening depression.

Attachment

the psychological connection between a child and his or her caretaker. Infants develop attachment behaviors within the first month. Deficits in early attachments can result in problems in later relationships in life.

Two recent reviews have focused on the issue of switching from depression into mania. In the first study reviewing a very complex literature on the subject using very sophisticated statistics, the switch rate appeared to be between 20% to 40%, with tricyclic antidepressants causing higher rates than SSRIs. The study also suggested that being on a mood stabilizer provided only partial protection against switching. In another study, however, which looked only at randomized trial data, switch rates on antidepressants were no different than placebo in the short run. Most agree that switching can definitely occur in patients with bipolar I disorder. The greatest controversy lies in how to properly treat patients with bipolar spectrum disorders, as the vast majority of them are predominantly depressed. Patients who are seen in a bipolar specialty clinic in a tertiary care center are less likely to be prescribed an antidepressant than if they saw a community psychiatrist. This may be due to the fact that most patients who are sent to a tertiary care center have already failed multiple medication trials, including antidepressants. In fact, it appears that one of the indicators of switching is a past history of failed multiple antidepressant trials. Finally, to complicate matters more, the abrupt withdrawal of antidepressant medications can cause a manic switch, so a slow taper is strongly advised for bipolar patients on them.

With respect to mood destabilization, or an increase in cycle frequency, the available literature seems to support the concept that the addition of antidepressants can cause patients to cycle much more often than if they were not on an antidepressant. Furthermore, bipolar disorder often worsens over the years through a process that may be identical to kindling (Question

27). Antidepressants may hasten the process, although there is no literature currently to support that. Unfortunately, no randomized studies have been performed, so the available literature is scant. Because studies have demonstrated reduced suicidality with patients on either Depakote (valproate) or lithium and no clear benefits with respect to suicidality with bipolar patients on antidepressants, most doctors feel strongly that treating depression with mood stabilizers that have antidepressant effects (lithium and Lamictal [lamotrigine]) should be the first course of action in bipolar patients, and if antidepressants are necessary they should be discontinued as soon as the depression has resolved.

A long history of research demonstrates a link between hormonal levels and mood disorders. Hormones are chemicals produced by **endocrine glands** that are released into the blood stream to carry out functions in other parts of the body. Hormone-producing endocrine glands include the thyroid, which produces thyroid hormone; the adrenal glands, which produce adrenaline or epinephrine, among others; and the reproductive glands, which produce testosterone and estrogen, among others. Hormones clearly play a role in various mood disorders such as premenstrual dysphoric disorder, postpartum depression, major depression, and bipolar disorder. Recently the issue of steroid use among professional athletes has been discussed in the press, as there have been a number of cases of suicides in previously mentally healthy young men who used them as performance enhancers (see Question 88). Steroids are often used to treat a variety of medical conditions that cause inflammation as they reduce the inflammatory process. But steroids are extremely activating, causing the body to mobilize into the "fight

Endocrine glands
ductless glands in the body that synthesize and secrete chemical messengers (hormones) into the blood stream or lymph for transport to target cells.

181

or flight" mode. The body also generates this mode naturally when very stressful circumstances occur. It is caused by a part of the involuntary, or autonomic, nervous system (see Question 3) known as the **sympathetic nervous system**. Its counterpoint, which causes "rest or restoration," is known as the **parasympathetic nervous system**. These systems act on both the body and the brain. The sympathetic system uses the chemical norepinephrine (noradrenalin), which is similar to epinephrine (adrenalin). Epinephrine is often given to people who have severe allergies to bee stings, foods, or medications. These allergic reactions cause a condition known as anaphylaxis, which can cause such severe swelling in the pharynx, making it impossible to breathe. Epinephrine is life saving in such circumstances. But the consequences are that the system is activated. For those with mood disorders, particularly bipolar disorder, this can have a destabilizing effect and cause relapse. Any medication that activates the sympathetic nervous system can do this, not just steroids. Medications used to treat asthma, emphysema, chronic bronchitis, or other pulmonary conditions that cause wheezing stimulate the sympathetic system to make the airways bigger in order to breathe easier. These medications are known as beta-agonists as they stimulate beta-receptors of the sympathetic nervous system, causing the airways to dilate. Such stimulation, however, affects the sympathetic nervous system throughout the body in addition to the airways.

There are also over-the-counter medications that can have a similar effect. Prior to removal from the market, Ephedra was known for this effect, but any medication that contains phenylpropanolamine has that potential. Stimulants, too, can potentially do this. The final com-

Sympathetic nervous system

the part of the autonomic nervous system that is responsible for providing responses and energy needed to cope with stressful situations such as fear or extremes of physical activity.

Parasympathetic nervous system

that part of the autonomic nervous system that allows for rest, recovery, and storage of new energy in the body between stressful situations.

mon pathway of all these medications, including anti-depressants, appears to be their impact on norepineph-rine, of which TCAs have more of an impact than SSRIs. But this includes street drugs that have stimu-lant properties or hallucinogenic properties (uppers and hallucinogens). Downers, on the other hand, which include barbiturates and alcohol, can destabilize mood due to their withdrawal effects, which mimic a sympathetic response. This is one of the reasons why it is critical to avoid alcohol and drugs of abuse. Finally, because of the popularity of recent herbal remedies, we have listed various herbs with psychotropic effects, with their adverse effects and interactions, in Table 6 (on page 117). These herbs should be avoided by all individuals with mood disorders.

84. Are there any medical conditions that can cause mania or depression?

Medical conditions should always be considered as a potential cause or exacerbating source for a manic or depressive episode. Because of their medical back-ground, psychiatrists routinely consider medical condi-tions as possible causes for mood disorders and thus will assess a person's medical history. Your psychiatrist may consider obtaining laboratory tests as part of screening for medical conditions, or he or she may defer this evaluation to your primary care physician. Most often, mania and depression occur independently of another medical disorder, but if there are physical signs and symptoms other than those typically found in a mood disorder, a medical/physical examination to rule out physical causes for the mood symptoms is war-ranted. Also, if a medical condition exists, it may very well be that the mood symptoms are not physiologically related but merely co-occurring with the illness.

Endocrine disorder

a disorder of the endocrine system. Endocrine glands release chemicals (also known as hormones), whose actions occur at another site, directly into the blood stream.

Endocrine disorders, cardiac conditions, cancers, neurological conditions, vitamin deficiencies, autoimmune disorders, and so on can be associated with depression or mania. Treatment of the co-occurring medical disorder may not result in resolution of the mood symptoms, but their resolution would support the physiological connection. Even so, for chronic medical conditions, long-term treatment may still be required with antidepressant or antimanic medications.

Table 8 lists medical conditions that can be associated with mania and depression. So-called secondary mania can occur from brain-based disorders, such as head injury, stroke, tumors, and migraines. Bipolar disorder is more common in patients with multiple sclerosis than in the general population. Infections that may result in mania include HIV, Lyme disease, and neurosyphilis.

Table 8   Medical causes of depression and mania

Medical Causes of Depression
Endocrine: hypothyroid, Cushing's disease, Addison's disease, diabetes
Infection: AIDS, Lyme disease, hepatitis
Cancer: pancreatic, occult, brain
Neurological: dementia, Parkinson's disease, stroke
Cardiac: coronary artery disease, heart failure, heart attack
Medications: antihypertensives, steroids, oral contraceptives

Medical Causes of Mania
Endocrine: hyperthyroid, Cushing's disease
Infection: AIDS, encephalitis, syphilis
Autoimmune: lupus
Neurological: multiple sclerosis, dementia, stroke, temporal lobe epilepsy
Medications: antidepressants, steroids, amphetamines, L-dopa

85. My aging father has always been an energetic individual but has never suffered from a mental illness. Recently he became manic for the first time in his life and ended up in the hospital. I had never heard of someone developing bipolar disorder in late life. Is that possible?

It is possible to develop bipolar disorder in late life. But it is important to distinguish between two types of mania in the geriatric population, primary mania and secondary mania. Primary mania is called bipolar disorder. Secondary mania is due to an underlying toxic or metabolic condition. About 10% of all patients with bipolar disorder have their first manic episode after the age of 50. However, both primary and secondary manias have a prevalence of less than 1% in the general geriatric population. In contrast to their younger peers, geriatric mania is usually associated with mixed manic and depressive symptoms and often associated with sleep disturbance, mood-incongruent paranoid delusions, cognitive impairments, and irritability more than hyperactivity. Additionally, increased goal-directed activities with a high degree of negative consequences are less prominent than in the younger population.

Distinguishing primary from secondary mania is of critical importance in this population, because underlying medical conditions associated with secondary mania often lead to **delirium** that comes with high mortality rates if the underlying medical condition is not corrected. Delirium is known also as an acute confusional state and is associated with a waxing and wan-

Delirium

a temporary state of mental confusion resulting from high fever, intoxication, shock, or other causes, and characterized by anxiety, disorientation, memory impairment, hallucinations, trembling, and incoherent speech.

ing of consciousness. Nighttime agitation and confusion, also known as "sun-downing," is more typically associated with delirium than primary mania. Neurological disorders are associated with about 75% of cases of secondary mania. These include encephalitis, other brain infections, vascula: diseases, tumors, and dementias. One must never leave out the prospect that the mania was medication induced. The geriatric population is particularly susceptible to medication side effects, and many medications can cause delirium and psychosis. Such medications include:

- Sedative/hypnotics (also alcohol)
- Anticholinergics (including Parkinson's disease medications and bladder control medications)
- Opiates (including Dilaudid or Fentanyl)
- Sympathomimetics (including decongestants, bronchodilators, and steroids)

The treatment for mania is symptom control, and therefore many of the treatments for primary and secondary mania are similar. Whenever a patient over the age of 50 with no prior history of mental illness presents with symptoms of mania, however, a thorough medical evaluation is indicated because the likelihood of an underlying medical condition causing the psychiatric symptoms increases dramatically with age. Thus the question of psychiatric treatment for primary verses secondary mania varies little in the acute phase of the illness. In the long run, however, patients with primary bipolar disorder will need to be maintained on their medication while those with secondary mania should be able to come off their psychiatric medications once the underlying medical condition is corrected.

86. I have sleep apnea in addition to bipolar disorder. What should I do?

The relation between bipolar disorder and insomnia is well established. During the manic phase of the illness, the resulting high energy leads to a decreased need for sleep. During the depressive phase, the reverse is often the case, with low energy and increased sleep, although in depression with typical vegetative symptoms, low energy is often associated with an inability to stay asleep, also known as middle insomnia. It is also well known that sleep deprivation can lead to or exacerbate an underlying mood disorder. Sleep deprivation can occur for many reasons. Anxiety in anticipation of an upcoming stressful event can often lead to trouble falling asleep and, if prolonged, could precipitate either a manic or depressive episode. Jet lag has also been known to precipitate mood disorders.

The most common causes of insomnia are medical causes. These causes are the most important to recognize and treat as these may not only precipitate a mood disorder but also render treatment of the mood disorder ineffective. Chief among these medical conditions is sleep apnea. Sleep apnea affects 2% of the 30- to 60-year-old male population and half as many of the female population. Apnea is defined as a cessation of breath that lasts at least ten seconds. Additionally there may be episodes known as **hypopnea**. This is defined as a significant reduction in airflow lasting at least ten seconds and usually associated with a decline in a person's oxygen level. People are considered to have sleep apnea if they have more than ten apneas and hypopneas per hour of sleep (commonly referred to as the apnea-hypopnea index, or AHI). This can only be diagnosed using a test known as polysomnography in a sleep lab. Polysomnography meas-

Hypopnea

abnormally slow, shallow breathing.

Special Populations

ures multiple factors associated with sleep, including brain waves through electroencephalography (EEG) that measure the various stages of sleep, respiratory rates and other vital signs, pulse oximetry that measures oxygenation, and motor activity.

Sleep apnea is generally classified into three types: central, obstructive, and mixed, with the latter two being much more common. Central sleep apnea occurs when the brain neglects to send signals to the chest muscles ordering them to breathe. Central sleep apnea is a neurological condition—there is no "mechanical" obstruction involved, as is the case with obstructive sleep apnea (OSA). OSA, the most common form of sleep apnea, occurs when a breathing effort is initiated but air is blocked from entering the lungs because the rear of the throat collapses and blocks the airway. Mixed apnea occurs when both central and obstructive elements are demonstrated by polysomnography. Thus there is limited or delayed inspiratory effort, and subsequently, when efforts are initiated the apnea persists because the upper airway is blocked. The consequence of sleep apnea is that sleep is disrupted with frequent awakenings that may not necessarily be perceived by the sleeper. Sleep is therefore of poor quality. The reason most people are not aware of this is because they do not fully wake up but instead spend an inordinate amount of time in Stage 1 light sleep and much less in Stage 3 or 4 (restful or deep sleep) and REM (dream) sleep. The result is that people complain of very poor sleep no matter how many hours they "sleep" in bed and feel they need to nap throughout the day. This not only leads to problems with mood but also can increase the risk of cardiac disease, affect memory, cause headaches, lead to weight gain, and cause impotency. Risk factors for sleep apnea include obesity (up to one-third of obese individuals have OSA), a large neck, recessed chin, male gender, structural abnormalities with the upper airway, smoking, and alcohol use. If your sleeping partner notices loud snoring followed by periods of silence, you should seek a medical evaluation for the condition. Risk factors also point to treatment. Weight loss and avoidance of alcohol and tobacco are the most obvious first-line approaches. An ear, nose, and throat doctor (also known as an otolaryngologist or ENT) evaluation may be indicated in order to determine if there is a structural abnormality that can be surgically repaired. Finally, continuous positive airway pressure, known as CPAP, is the treatment of choice. This includes a pump and a mask that essentially forces the airway open to allow more ease of breathing. Patients often initially complain of the mask and noise associated with this treatment and, as a result, compliance is often a problem. However, with time one can adjust to these initial difficulties. The results CPAP provides in terms or morbidity and mortality are well worth the effort.

Scott's comments:
I was recently diagnosed with sleep apnea. My prescribed treatment was CPAP, and I've been on CPAP therapy now for about 3–4 months. My moods are now more stable, as I've not been sleep deprived. I found that the CPAP therapy can help return my general mood to a baseline that is closer to my perception of "normal."

87. What is the relation between thyroid problems and bipolar disorder?

Thyroid dysfunction is associated with mood disorders with symptoms of hypothyroidism able to mimic depression and of hyperthyroidism able to mimic mania. People with an overactive thyroid may exhibit marked anxiety and tension, emotional lability, impatience and irritability, distractible overactivity, exaggerated sensitivity to noise, and fluctuating depression with sadness as well as problems with sleep and the appetite. In extreme cases psychosis can develop. Cases of hyperthyroidism-induced mania are rare, however. People with underactive thyroid may exhibit depressed mood, anxiety, inattentiveness, slowing of thought, weakness, poor memory, and sleep difficulties with psychosis in more extreme cases. Again, the incidence of thyroid dysfunction in depressed patients is low, more likely being present in treatment-resistant depression. It has been postulated that a surplus of thyroid hormone could lead to mania by promoting the action of catecholamines at central receptor sites, and, conversely, low thyroid levels could diminish the use of norepinephrine in times of stress, leading to depression. Tests for thyroid dysfunction should be given, as it is simple to test and if present, treatment of the thyroid dysfunction may resolve the mood disorder.

People with bipolar disorder often have abnormal thyroid gland function, with women more likely to be afflicted than men. Because too much or too little thyroid hormone alone can lead to mood and energy changes, thyroid levels should be carefully monitored by a physician. Interestingly, a high prevalence of thyroid hypofunction has been found in bipolar patients, being estimated to occur in almost one out of every ten bipolar patients not being treated with certain mood-stabilizing medications (that cause thyroid dysfunction). Although not common, there have been cases of mania reported secondary to hypothyroidism as well. Several studies have shown a higher incidence of hypothyroidism in patients with rapid-cycling bipolar disorder than in nonrapid cyclers. Thyroid treatment of hypothyroidism in rapid cyclers has been shown to decrease the severity and frequency of manic and depressive episodes, and high-dose thyroid hormone has been used to treat refractory rapid cycling in the absence of measurable thyroid deficiency. Hypothyroidism may induce or contribute to the induction of rapid cycling in bipolar illness.

Long-term lithium use can cause hypothyroid function, which may account for some depressive episodes that occur during treatment. This is usually reversible unless antithyroid antibodies have developed. Lithium-induced thyroid dysfunction is more likely to occur in women. Treatment with lithium is often continued with thyroid supplementation provided.

88. I was put on steroids for treatment of a medical condition. I ended up in the emergency room after several sleepless nights, confused, disoriented, and hallucinating. I was given an anti-psychotic medication and was told that I needed to keep taking it because I was bipolar. I have never had a mental illness in my life. Was it just due to the steroids, or do I now have a new condition?

Steroids make up a large family of chemical compounds including hormones, body constituents, and drugs such as sterols, cardiac glycosides, androgens, estrogens, corticosteroids, bile acids, sterols, and precursors of vitamin D and cholesterol. Almost no function in the body occurs without the involvement of one of these compounds. Most steroids prescribed as medicine are used to reduce inflammation. Inflammation causes pain and swelling and can lead to other symptoms as well. Allergic reactions, autoimmune diseases, or other inflammatory diseases such as chronic obstructive pulmonary disease or emphysema are treated with steroids in order to reduce their symptoms.

Steroids have multiple effects on the body aside from their anti-inflammatory effects. They can cause the "fight or flight" response through activation of the sympathetic nervous system, as mentioned in Question 82. This effect causes various physiological changes in the body such as an increase in blood flow to the muscles, an increase in heart rate and blood pressure, and a state of hyper-alertness. This hyper-alertness can have psychiatric effects: from a general fear response to frank paranoia including delusions and hallucinations, insomnia, and mood swings from depression to mania. Prednisone is the most commonly prescribed medication in this family, and the psychiatric effects appear to be based on three factors: the dose, the change in rate of the dose over time, and finally the length of time receiving the medication. Euphoria and anxiety tend to be the most common mild psychiatric side effects followed by frank mania and depression, with depression more common upon rapid withdrawal of the medication. Studies have shown that in patients with no psychiatric history, measuring only severe psychiatric disturbances resulting from prednisone found a rate of about 2%, with increasing rates to as high as 20% as dosage increases. Some of the most commonly known names of corticosteroids include:

- Cortisone and Hydrocortisone
- Flonase

- Lanacort
- Prednisone
- Nasonex

Corticosteroids are used in the treatment of a variety of medical conditions including:

- Asthma
- Emphysema
- Crohn's disease
- Bursitis
- Tendonitis
- Ulcerative colitis
- Hives
- Insect bites
- Nasal allergies
- Eczema
- Psoriasis

The management of steroid-induced mania and/or psychosis is the same as if one had bipolar disorder, which includes both mood-stabilizing medication and/or antipsychotic medication. No evidence currently supports the notion that chronic steroid use causes bipolar disorder; however, there are cases of steroids unmasking a previously undiagnosed bipolar disorder. How often this happens is unclear but it is much rarer than steroid-induced mania or psychosis. The difference between these two conditions is more in terms of the difference in the length of time one needs to be on psychotropic medication. If the condition is merely steroid induced it will eventually resolve with the discontinuation of steroids, and the patient will be able to come off psychotropic medication as well. If it is bipolar disorder, eliminating the steroids will not eliminate the underlying condition and long-term psychotropic medication will be necessary. If you have steroid-induced mania or bipolar disorder it is critical to inform the doctor the next time you require steroid treatment. Studies have shown that adequate **prophylaxis** with a mood stabilizer or antipsychotic can prevent future episodes.

Prophylaxis

the prevention of disease.

PART VII

Surviving

What are my rights to refuse hospitalization?

What are my rights to refuse medication and other treatments?

What are my rights to privacy?

More ...

89. What are my rights to refuse hospitalization?

The right to refuse hospitalization varies from state to state. That being said, most states have fairly similar criteria for involuntary hospitalization or what is also known as civil commitment. Such criteria are that a mental illness is present and the person is imminently dangerous to self or others. Ways in which the criteria may differ from state to state are primarily on the length of stay allowed prior to court review and on minor procedural differences. There may also be differences as to whether inclusion of a term called *grave disability* can be added as an additional criterion when deciding to hospitalize an individual involuntarily. Some states do not allow for this. The designation of grave disability means an individual is so disabled by a mental illness that he or she is in imminent danger due to the disability. For example, an individual with severe diabetes who has stopped taking insulin because of severe depression would be considered in grave danger of developing a diabetic coma.

Some historical background is helpful in order to understand the basis of one's rights to refuse hospitalization. Involuntary commitment to a psychiatric hospital was first based upon the legal term *parens patriae* (Latin for "parent of his country"). Under this doctrine, the state or government, as represented by a physician, acted as the "parent" for the mentally ill individual and could commit him or her to a psychiatric facility merely based on the opinion that the patient was in need of such care. A landmark 1973 case, *Lessard vs. Schmidt*, in Wisconsin changed this law. Alberta Lessard, the plaintiff, was involuntarily committed and argued successfully that her rights were violated because of that commitment. First, she argued that the grounds upon which she was committed, parens patriae law, was overly vague by defining a mentally ill individual as one who requires care and treatment for his own welfare or for the welfare of others in the community. Second, she argued that the procedure used to commit her violated her civil rights by denying her due process. The court agreed on both counts arguing that the patient had all the rights accorded to a criminal suspect. As a result of this case, parens patriae was replaced by the requirement that an individual meet the criteria of being both mentally ill and imminently dangerous in order to be involuntarily committed. The courts hoped to decrease the number of admissions to psychiatric hospitals by defining the commitment standards more narrowly, as they considered such action as potentially more damaging than the risks to the individual and community by not committing them.

A second legal ruling occurred in 1976, known as the **Tarasoff** case, after the family of a girl murdered by a man sued for not being warned of the man's threats to murder the girl. The man had told his psychologist of his intentions and the psychologist notified the police of the man's threats. The police performed their own interview of the man. Based on their interview there was no evidence that the man was either mentally ill or imminently dangerous and he was released. The initial court ruling held that both the police and the treating clinicians were responsible, but on appeal the case against the police was dropped while the clinicians were held to an even greater standard that required of them the duty to protect. With the growing concern about the increasing liability one accepts for treating

Tarasoff

the name of a family that sued the therapist involved in the care of a young man who murdered a family member. As a result of the lawsuit, therapists are now required to protect and warn potential victims from violent acts or threats made by patients under their care.

individuals with potential for such acts, and the fact that there is no science to predict dangerousness, the number of individuals involuntarily committed has skyrocketed, leading to a consequence the courts hoped to actually avert.

Understanding the history behind involuntary commitment is important to understand the right to refuse hospitalization. Expressing suicidal or homicidal feelings does not automatically mandate immediate hospitalization. Consideration is given to what is said, how it is said, and to whom it is said. The less the clinician knows the patient, the more careful that clinician will be in asking further questions or in referring the patient to an emergency room to be evaluated for hospitalization. Nothing regarding safety is taken lightly under these circumstances, even if one is expressing feelings in a way that he or she believes is figurative and not literal. It is important to have a strong, trusting relationship with one's treating clinician where all options for treatment can be discussed openly and freely without fear. Under those circumstances hospitalization may be raised as an option among many others for thorough discussion. The clinician should be able to describe parameters for when hospitalization is considered an absolute necessity. The clinician may ask for outside supports such as family members to be more involved in order to avoid hospitalization. In fact, an adequate support system is one of the single most critical factors in maintaining safety and avoiding hospitalization.

Patients who are hospitalized involuntarily have options available to appeal the commitment. The right to due process and legal representation is maintained. Depending on the state, this may include a court-appointed attorney or a legal advocate. A specific time limit is usually set by the state within which a patient has a legal right to have a hearing before a judge to request release from the hospital. Hospitals are also required to post a patient's "bill of rights" and hand them out to every patient. Even when involuntarily committed, patients continue to have the right to refuse treatment and cannot be medicated without consent unless there is a clear and immediate danger toward self or others. Legally known as a chemical restraint, this is typically a one-time dose of a short-acting medication to help calm the patient. Physical restraint or seclusion may also be applied to prevent a patient from harming one's self or others. The federal government mandates specific requirements regarding the application of such restraints, including appropriate monitoring and documentation of restraint usage, and specific time limits within which reevaluation by a physician is required.

90. What are my rights to refuse medication and other treatments?

Unlike involuntary hospitalization where issues of safety trump autonomy, the right to refuse treatment continues to be sacrosanct (except as noted in Question 89 regarding the use of "chemical restraints"). In general, patients have the absolute right to refuse medical or psychiatric treatment of any kind, short of emergency hospitalization for issues of safety. The clinician must obtain **informed consent** prior to prescribing any treatment. Informed consent is a legal and ethical doctrine fundamental to modern medicine. The process of obtaining informed consent includes the following elements:

Informed consent
the premise that patients have a right to determine what happens to their body, and as such agreement to a treatment requires receipt of information, competence to make the decision, and agreeability for the treatment.

- Assessment of the patient's capacity to make medical decisions
- Absence of coercion of the patient
- Patient is fully informed of his or her diagnosis and prognosis, risks versus benefits of the treatment offered, risks versus benefits of alternative treatments, and risks versus benefits of receiving no treatment

There are few but notable exceptions to informed consent. These exceptions include emergencies, therapeutic privilege, therapeutic waiver, and implied consent. In many emergency situations the patient is unconscious and in need of life-saving treatment. Informed consent is assumed or obtained to the best of the clinician's ability. When clinicians assume therapeutic privilege, they are withholding information from the patient because they believe informing the patient will cause more harm than good. Occasionally patients will request not to be informed. In other words, they waive their right to be informed. Such a waiver is not advisable. One should enlist the aid of a family member to make decisions when one wants to remove oneself from the decision. Finally, implied consent occurs when one offers one's arm to have blood drawn or his or her blood pressure checked.

When refusing medication or treatment, it is important to be informed of and understand the potential consequences of refusing. Understanding the consequences requires one to have the capacity to refuse treatment. Capacity to refuse treatment requires four elements:

- The ability to express a choice
- The ability to understand the treatment options and their consequences

- The ability to appreciate the information as it applies to one's specific situation
- The ability to reason with the information

All four elements must be met for a patient to have the capacity to decide upon medical or psychiatric treatment. Obviously most of these elements are generally understood between the patient and the clinician in most treatment decisions. These become important to sort out more clearly when someone is in a life-threatening situation and is refusing a life-saving treatment. Under those circumstances, a physician may call in a psychiatrist to evaluate one's capacity to refuse treatment, and if one lacks such capacity, he or she will recommend emergency conservatorship in order to help make such decisions. Usually a family member is appointed conservator under those circumstances.

There are fewer, though real, life-threatening psychiatric conditions even after someone has been hospitalized. The most obvious is when a patient remains out of control behaviorally and requires a chemical restraint. Less obvious is a patient so severely depressed he or she is no longer eating or drinking and is refusing all treatment. Under these circumstances, in most states a conservatorship hearing will only allow for medical treatments to maintain the person's life but will not allow for the administration of psychiatric treatment if that individual continues to refuse that form of care. In fact conservators generally only have the right to make decisions about medical care, housing, and finances. Conservators cannot sign someone into a psychiatric hospital and they cannot agree to have a person forcibly medicated. Instead a second hearing must occur during which independent psychiatrists review the case and report their findings to the court. Only then will a judge determine whether or not a person can receive psychiatric care against his or her will in the form of medication or some other therapy. This procedure typically occurs after a patient is hospitalized but continues to refuse medication. Under such circumstances the hospital pursues this course of action because it is believed the patient's health and well-being depend on treatment.

As an outpatient, you must understand and weigh the treatment options to the best of your ability and enlist outside support from other informative sources if needed. The right to refuse medication as an outpatient is respected most of the time. In fact, few states allow for involuntary outpatient treatment. This is changing, though in very specific and limited circumstances. Recent high-profile cases in various states where noncompliant mentally ill patients have injured or killed someone have prompted new involuntary outpatient treatment laws. But the requirements imposed upon caregivers for making their case for involuntary treatment are exceedingly stringent and require regular court review.

91. What are my rights to privacy?

Confidentiality has become one of the hottest issues in medicine in the past few years with the introduction of the new federal laws encompassed under the acronym HIPAA (for Health Insurance Portability and Accountability Act). The field of medicine has always regarded confidentiality as one of its highest ethical principles. Psychiatry has put even greater restrictions on confidentiality given the highly sensitive nature of the issues patients discuss. As a result no information is released to anyone without a written authorization by the patient allowing for such release. A written authorization for release of general medical records is not enough. The patient must knowingly and specifically request psychiatric and/or drug and alcohol information to be released before it can be. Every effort is made to protect a patient's right to privacy.

There are, however, exceptions to that right and it behooves everyone to know just what those exceptions are. First, confidentiality does not apply when a patient is considered to be a threat to others, unless hospitalized. Second, confidentiality does not apply when the law requires mandatory reporting. This includes communicable diseases, child or elder abuse, impaired driving, and any other requirement in a particular jurisdiction. Third, court-ordered or subpoenaed records can be released without the patient's written authorization. However, a good clinician will usually notify the patient and attempt to obtain written authorization before honoring the court's request. Fourth, hospitals and offices may release health care information without the patient's written permission for the purposes of treatment, payment, or operations (TPO), such as quality control, peer review, teaching, and so on. This is encompassed under the HIPAA rules. The most important factor to bear in mind when a clinician releases psychiatric information about a patient to another person without that patient's consent is the concept of "duty to third parties." Most lawyers would prefer to defend a breach of confidentiality case than a wrongful death case. Clinicians understand this all too well, and in emergency situations may feel obligated to violate a patient's autonomy and confidentiality in order to protect him or her and the community from some greater harm. This is especially true if the patient is being evaluated in an emergency room. In those instances clinicians will generally not feel comfortable discharging a patient before obtaining outside sources of information, and refusing to allow such contact will only delay discharge and probably ensure hospitalization under an involuntary commitment. Good clinicians, however, will always inform the patient of their decisions and whom they are contacting.

The initial impetus behind HIPAA was to extend the ability of people to maintain their health care insurance after termination of employment and decrease the exclusions for preexisting conditions. HIPAA was also an attempt by the government to provide further controls over fraud and abuse of the Medicare system. To most people, however, HIPAA has become synonymous with privacy because one of the first orders of business when one enters a doctor's office today is to receive a notice of privacy and sign that one received such notice. The notice of privacy outlines the various ways in which one's health care information can be shared without requiring written permission unless the person objects to any such release in writing beforehand, as outlined earlier. Again, the notice also outlines the release of health care information as mandated by law as pointed out previously. Additionally, it specifically mentions that psychiatric and drug and alcohol information are specially protected, though limited amounts of information on these diagnoses may be shared for the purposes of TPO. The notice specifically states that unless provided a written request it is assumed information such as appointments can be shared via phone, mail, or with family members, and so on. Finally, patients have the right to view and amend their health care information by submitting a written request. This right can be denied under specific circumstances outlined in the notice, but the patient has a right to know the reasons and may appeal such denials.

Generally, when you first enter a doctor's office and begin filling out a myriad of forms, one form will be to authorize release of information for purposes of treatment, payment, and operations. With respect to payment, your health insurance company requires medical information for the purposes of payment because they want to know what they are paying for. The term insurance companies use to authorize payment is *medical necessity*. This means that they want proof that the bill sent to them for a particular service was medically necessary and therefore deserving of payment. This also means that the clinician must send the insurer the diagnosis and the treatment rendered in order to demonstrate medical necessity. If a patient refuses to allow the release of such information, either the clinician may refuse to see or treat the patient or, if seen, the patient will be responsible for the bill.

92. Is it necessary to involve my family in my treatment?

Although the decision as to the level of involvement of a family member in the evaluation and treatment of bipolar disorder is generally up to you, your clinician may request (and in certain circumstances insist) that an involved family member be brought in as part of the evaluation process. Both mania and depression typically affect a person's cognitive abilities and can be so severe that the ability to make decisions becomes impaired. The involvement of a family member helps to clarify symptoms, relationship and work difficulties, as well as family history. The involved family member may have certain insights as to recent stressors that triggered the onset of the episode. Most important, your family can be a source of support during the initial phase of treatment and the recovery process. Due to effects on motivation, self-esteem, and feelings of self-sufficiency, a depressed or manic person may not engage fully in the treatment process. You may need reminders to take your medication and keep appointments. In particular, during the hypomanic or manic state, you may find it difficult to follow up in treatment, as this state is often one of good feeling. Affected individuals often do not recognize the symptoms in themselves, which is where family involvement becomes especially important. In addition, if you have suicidal thinking, an involved family member may be an important factor your clinician uses in determining your ability to be safe. A family member can monitor for suicidal behaviors. A person who is alone and without any support network is at higher risk for complications of bipolar disorder, including suicide. Thus, a clinician may insist a family member be involved in the treatment if it is believed your personal safety is at risk.

Leslie's comments:

For me, there was never a question whether to involve my partner in my treatment. After having suffered the consequences of living with me in an unmedicated state for many years, I believe it is only fair and right to be honest and upfront about my treatment. I think it would also do us both a huge disservice if I neglected to tell my partner about changes in my mood or to reject the feedback I get from her regarding any mood fluctuations she may witness. We are able to keep the consequences of the illness in check because we are both vigilant about the destructive power of the disorder and, in the meantime, are respectful of each other as well.

93. I'm worried about my employer finding out about my treatment.

All employees need to know that they are under *no* obligation to disclose medical information, whether they are seeking employment or are currently employed. Many job application forms request information about mental illness, and employers may request information about a gap in employment. Because many employers pay the medical bills, they frequently feel that they have a right to know an employee's medical history. If treatment requires time away from work, some medical information may need to be released in order to justify the time off.

The information given to an employer is strictly at the employee's discretion. If information is shared with the employer by a health care professional or a health care institution without the patient's permission, legal sanctions may be invoked that will penalize the provider for releasing confidential information. The threat of legal sanctions should prevent the employer from finding out about your health status. The legal sanctions are described in the previous question about "your right to privacy."

Many patients fear that if an employer finds out about their history of bipolar disorder they will be fired. The American Disabilities Act (ADA) is a federal law that was passed to protect patients with disabilities from being fired because of a specific disability. The ADA of 1990 makes it unlawful to discriminate against an employee if he or she is a qualified individual with a disability. A disabled individual is defined as "a person who has a physical or mental impairment that substantially limits one or more major life activities, has a record of such impairment or is regarded as having such impairment" (U.S. Equal Employment Opportunity Commission, 1991). This law also applies to people with mental disorders, including bipolar disorder. If the disabled person is the most qualified person among all of the applicants to do the job then accommodations must be made, such as job restructuring, modifying work schedules, and acquiring or modifying equipment. According to the ADA, employers cannot discriminate in their hiring and firing practices based on medical information, which includes psychiatric information. Such discrimination is considered a violation of the ADA law. The law specifically prohibits an employer from asking questions about a person's disability during an employee's job interview unless the questions are directly related to job requirements. The same principle holds true once the prospective employee is hired. The bottom line: current laws protect employees from unwanted disclosures to employers, which should prevent the employer from finding out about your bipolar disorder. In this case, the law is on your side in preventing your employer from finding out about your medical status.

94. Will I get manic or depressed again after I have recovered?

Bipolar disorder is generally an episodic, lifelong illness with a variable course. The risk for becoming depressed or manic again in the future is high, with higher risk for recurrent depression. Although early in the disease episodes may occur far apart in time, as years go by, episodes frequently become closer together. This may be due in part to brain changes that occur during each episode. Thus, it is important to prevent as many episodes as possible. With untreated bipolar disorder, ten or more episodes may occur over a person's lifetime. In contrast to major depressive disorder, for which consideration can be given to stop medication, the recommendation for an episode of mania is to continue medication, due to the high risk for a future episode of depression or mania. Ongoing studies are looking at the maintenance treatment of bipolar disorder and the effect of medication on decreasing episodes of depression and/or mania. Most medications approved in the treatment of bipolar disorder have not been adequately studied for their ability to prevent relapse. At present, Lamictal (lamotrigine) has FDA approval for prevention of recurrence of depressive episodes. Maintenance treatment with lithium and Depakote has been shown to lower the risk for suicide in bipolar patients.

The medication regimen that successfully treated the acute manic episode should typically be continued in the maintenance phase. Often more than one medication is required for stabilization. Sometimes, efforts to reduce medication dosage or cut back to one medication are made during the maintenance phase, but there is evidence that doing so may increase the risk for relapse. In a recent two-year-long, multi-center study, published in 2006 in the *American Journal of Psychiatry*, close to 50% of patients relapsed. The mean time to recurrence was ~ 45 weeks. Two-thirds of the recurrences were depressive episodes and one-third were manic or hypomanic episodes. Residual depressive and manic symptoms were significantly associated with risk of recurrence. This study demonstrated that the maintenance treatment of bipolar disorder still requires ongoing investigation.

The goals of maintenance treatment in bipolar disorder are relapse prevention, reduction of subthreshold symptoms, and reduction of suicide risk, as well as reduction of cycling frequency and mood instability, and improvement of functioning.

95. What can I do if I have failed several forms of medication and therapy?

Unfortunately there are situations when bipolar disorder does not respond to conventional treatments available. This can be frustrating and certainly contributes to the morbidity of bipolar disorder. Sometimes it can be helpful to obtain a consultation by a different clinician to examine your treatment history and perhaps make some other suggestions. A lack of response to treatment might be due to inadequate dosing or duration of medication trials, or due to a missed diagnosis. Comorbid conditions can make a bipolar illness more refractory to treatment. Conditions that may co-occur with bipolar disorder include anxiety disorders (panic disorder, generalized anxiety disorder, obsessive-compulsive disorder, social anxiety disorder), posttraumatic stress disorder (also an anxiety condition), attention-deficit disorder, and substance abuse disorders. Further evaluation and treatment of other conditions may be necessary. Substance abuse treatment, for example, may need to be obtained in order for the bipolar condition to be adequately treated. Sometimes a refractory major depression is a missed bipolar depression, so careful reevaluation may be needed in this case as well. Psychiatrists use guidelines in the treatment of **refractory depression** and recurrent mania. Often, different medication combinations have yet to be tried, and

Refractory depression

depressive illness that does not respond to a therapeutic intervention. The term is not typically applied unless such a lack of response has occurred to several different interventions.

ECT may need consideration as well. Although all psychiatrists are trained in psychopharmacologic treatments, some individuals have a specific expertise in the field of psychopharmacology for bipolar disorder. These individuals are typically associated with an academic institution, so that is a potential referral source. In addition, there are usually research protocols being conducted in association with academic institutions investigating newer medications. Participation in a research protocol usually involves a comprehensive evaluation during which other diagnostic possibilities are investigated as well.

96. What is the risk of suicide when someone is diagnosed with bipolar disorder?

The overall mortality rate of bipolar disorder is two to three times higher than in the general population. About 10% to 20% of bipolar individuals commit suicide, and upward to one-third admit to at least one suicide attempt. The third with a history of suicide attempts have a number of additional risk factors. These risk factors include a family history of drug abuse and suicide (or attempts), a greater personal history of early traumatic stressors such as sexual and physical abuse, more hospitalizations for depression, a course of increasing severity of mania, more Axis I, II, and III conditions, and more time ill overall. Bipolar individuals with a history of suicide attempts experience more episodes of depression and react to them by having severe suicidal ideation. They demonstrate behaviorally an overall higher level of lifetime aggression and a pattern of repeated suicide attempts.

Surviving

In addition, mania decreases impulse control. A person with mixed mania and depression is at an even higher risk of suicide attempts because he or she is generally irritable, dysphoric, anxious, energized, *and* behaviorally disinhibited. A person with poor impulse control may be more apt to attempt suicide because the time interval between the thought and the act can be instantaneous. Anyone with plans to kill him- or herself, or who has made an attempt, requires emergency psychiatric evaluation. In some situations, a family member finds out that someone has tried to kill him- or herself but does not take him or her to an emergency room because of assurances to the family member that it was a mistake and that he or she will be okay. It is best, however, if a professional evaluates the situation to determine the most appropriate course of action.

Suicide is the most serious risk of bipolar disorder. Clinicians assess suicide risk based on many factors, including the patient's current mental status, personal history, family history, use of substances, and more. Suicidal thinking tends to fall on a continuum from morbid thoughts of death to passive thoughts of wishing to be dead to an actual plan to carry out the suicide, a continuum that is assessed by the clinician. Clinicians will ask direct questions about suicidal thoughts. Direct questions do not put ideas in a person's mind; rather, they invite the individual to speak openly about the issue. Most patients want help and want to let someone know how they are feeling. Also in this light, if you have reason to believe a family member is contemplating suicide, it is best to speak openly and frankly to that person about your concerns. Doing so will not put new thoughts of suicide into the person's mind; instead, it will give an opportunity to help him or her get the treatment that may be needed.

97. A family member committed suicide. I feel guilty that I missed something.

Suicide is the single most tragic outcome of patients suffering from mental illness. No matter how prepared someone thinks he or she is that a family member may eventually commit suicide because of his or her pain and suffering, it always feels unexpected and comes as a complete surprise. When it happens, everyone, including family, friends, and caregivers, feels shocked. Some are completely devastated with guilt about the loss. Small, seemingly insignificant events leading up to the person's death, appearing at the time to be normal, take on a new and painful meaning in retrospect. These events evolve into clear signs of the person's commitment to the inevitable last act, thus heightening the feelings of guilt. There may be a sense of having let the person down, of saying the wrong thing, or not being there when he or she needed you most. When looked at in retrospect, everyone asks himself or herself, "How could I have missed that?" These are perfectly normal feelings.

An exact science of predicting suicide is not presently established and probably never will be established. There are people who live their lives with chronic suicidal ideation and never act on their thoughts. There are people who engage in countless acts of cutting and overdosing without any significant physical harm to themselves. Alternatively, there are people who never think of suicide their entire lives until the moment they commit suicide. Despite the advances psychiatry has made in assessing and treating mental illness, it is only one of many risk factors that contribute to suicide. Epidemiologists develop risk factors by looking at population aggregates of people who attempt or complete suicide and establishing the frequency that various factors correlate with suicide. But correlation does not mean causation. Although risk factors can help to assess someone who is at risk for suicide, they play little role in helping to predict if and when a person at risk will attempt or complete suicide. As a result, psychiatry is an inexact science at best, and the ability to predict suicide is worse than forecasting the weather. One can never underestimate the power of free will. Although guilt is a feeling one cannot control and is often a normal expected response under such circumstances, one is rarely guilty for another's actions.

98. My son keeps going off his medication. He ends up back in the hospital and they keep him there for only a week or so before letting him out again. I am frustrated and angry. He needs long-term hospitalization. How can I get him that level of care?

The term *noncompliance* refers to a patient voluntarily stopping treatment against his or her physician's recommendations. There are several reasons why noncompliance occurs. The most common reason is a failure to recognize that one has bipolar disorder. The second most common reason for noncompliance is having a personality disorder and/or an ongoing drug and alcohol problem. Additional reasons for noncompliance are listed in Table 9. Other reasons that make compliance difficult include the number of medica-

Table 9

Reasons for treatment noncompliance
Failure to recognize one has bipolar disorder
Comorbid personality disorder
Ongoing drug and/or alcohol problem
Fear of being labeled "crazy"
Loss of the euphoria
Fear of losing one's creativity or personality
A belief one has been cured
Desire for more "natural remedies"
Medication side effects
Forgetfulness or loss of motivation due to depression
Cost of medication
Lack of access to health care and medication

tions one is taking and the number of health care providers one is seeing who are prescribing medications. Once per day dosing is available for some medications and thus may improve compliance. Many medications have interactions, which further complicates matters because the interactions can lead to either increased side effects or loss of effectiveness. It is important to know the underlying reason and address it immediately to improve compliance.

Noncompliance in bipolar disorder reaches 66% and is the single biggest reason for relapse and rehospitalization, homelessness, and legal problems. The common denominator underpinning many of these reasons is the physician-patient relationship. In countries where respect for the physician's authority remains high and relationships between physicians and patients develop over the years, rates of compliance are higher even when the patient denies having an illness. The critical factor is finding a physician who is able, available, and affable (the 3 A's of a good physician). An able physician not only understands the research and complexity of psychiatric diagnoses and medications but also is capable of explaining that complexity in a manner that is simple and straightforward so that all the risks and benefits of being on or off the medications are clearly outlined. An available physician not only allows for timely appointments with adequate time during appointments but is also flexible with his or her time and can make time for urgent needs as well as urgent phone calls. An affable physician is warm and empathic, never arrogant or condescending. There are a lot of unknowns in medicine in general and psychiatry in particular. A good physician is one who admits ignorance and is willing to do the research to answer questions that he or she may not have immediate knowledge of at the time.

Finding a willing physician with the above qualities is the start of providing help to a family member developing compliance. Toward that end, becoming educated about bipolar disorder will help to develop realistic expectations and coping mechanisms for when things go wrong. Review "worst case scenarios" so that a crisis plan can be established. Instability is typically the rule at first because it is often very difficult to find the right medication or combination of medications that achieve stability without significant side effects. During this time it is easy to become frustrated and discouraged. Frequent hospitalizations may occur and a lot of angry words can be exchanged between patient and family during this period. Educate and involve everyone in the family to improve the support system, which improves the odds of success. Everyone should know about the medications and their side effects, names of the health care providers and how to contact them, and even attend some appointments together. Openness in communication is imperative. Bipolar disorder should be treated as you would treat any other medical condition. That means while a certain amount of respect for privacy should be maintained, issues of health, disability, or safety involve the whole family. Avoid health care providers who are unwilling to talk to family members and who hide under the old guise of psychotherapeutic privilege. This approach may be fine for the "worried well" patients, but for patients suffering from bipolar disorder it is generally the wrong approach to take. Family therapy can be useful toward that end. Getting involved with the local chapter of the National Alliance for the Mentally Ill (NAMI) to improve the support system available is also recommended.

Long-term hospitalization, for all intents and purposes, no longer exists, particularly for patients suffering from bipolar disorder. The seriously mentally ill have been increasingly cared for, supported, and treated in the community, with brief crisis hospitalizations occurring at local hospitals. The average length of stay, depending upon the geographic region, ranges from three to fourteen days with better than 90% of discharges occurring within the first five to seven days. The purpose of these hospitalizations is primarily to reduce the risk of dangerousness or disability to a level that can generally be managed safely in the community. For most family members, this is generally a frustrating experience because their loved ones are usually still symptomatic. While you may disagree with the many ethical, social, and economic reasons for why this way of caring for the mentally ill occurs, it remains the current system of care. For this reason you must ensure the highest level of support is obtained in the community in order to achieve the highest level of success. Toward that end, the local chapter of NAMI often becomes a repository for resource acquisition, and you should call upon it immediately to know what is available in your community.

99. What is NAMI? How can they help?

NAMI is an acronym for the National Alliance for the Mentally Ill, an advocacy group made up predominantly of family members of patients and patients themselves suffering from mental illness. As its mission statement reports: "NAMI is dedicated to the eradication of mental illnesses and to the improvement of the quality of life of all those whose lives are affected by these diseases." From its inception in 1979 NAMI has worked very hard to advocate for the mentally ill in order to achieve equitable services and treatment for more than fifteen million patients and their families in need. It is an all-volunteer organization with more than a thousand local chapters in all fifty states that provides education to consumers and the community, lobby for increased research, and provides advocacy for health insurance, housing, rehabilitation, and jobs for those struggling with mental illness. As each community has unique characteristics and needs, each chapter serves to meet these needs on an individual community basis. There is a website, *www.nami.org*, that can provide further information and resources for those interested in becoming involved in their local chapters.

100. Where can I find out more information about bipolar disorder?

It is not possible to discuss all aspects of bipolar disorder in one small volume. In Appendix A that follows there is information on organizations, websites, and publications that can be useful to patients with bipolar disorder and their families.

Surviving

Appendix A

Resources

Organizations

American Foundation for Suicide Prevention
120 Wall Street, 22nd Floor
New York, NY 10005
(888) 333-AFSP
www.afsp.org

Child and Adolescent Bipolar Foundation
1000 Skokie Blvd., Suite 570
Wilmette, IL 60091
www.bpkids.org

Depression and Bipolar Support Alliance
730 N. Franklin Street, Suite 501
Chicago, IL 60610-7224
(800) 826-3632
www.dbsalliance.org

Depression and Related Affective Disorders Association
2330 West Joppa Rd.
Suite 100
Lutherville, MD 21093
(410) 583-2919
www.drada.org

Families for Depression Awareness
300 Fifth Avenue
Waltham, MA 02451
(781) 890-0220
www.familyaware.org

National Alliance for the Mentally Ill
Colonial Place Three
2107 Wilson Blvd., Suite 300
Arlington, VA 22201-3042
(703) 524-7600
www.nami.org

National Institute of Mental Health
Office of Communications
6001 Executive Boulevard, Room 8184, MSC 9663
Bethesda, MD 20892-9663
(301) 443-4513
www.nimh.nih.gov

National Mental Health Association
2001 N. Beauregard Street, 12th Floor
Alexandria, VA 22311
(800) 969-NMHA
www.nmha.org

Food and Drug Administration
5600 Fishers Lane
Rockville, Maryland 20857
(888) INFO-FDA
www.fda.gov

Hotline Numbers

National Adolescent Suicide Hotline
(800) 621-4000

National Drug and Alcohol Treatment Hotline
(800) 662-HELP

National Suicide Prevention Lifeline
(800) 273-TALK

National Youth Crisis Hotline
(800) HIT-HOME

Websites

www.aabt.org
Association for Advancement of Behavior Therapy website with
  link to find a therapist

www.aacap.org
American Academy of Child and Adolescent Psychiatry website
  with resources for patients and their families

www.aboutourkids.org
NYU Child Study Center website on child mental health

www.academyofct.org
The Academy of Cognitive Therapy website with links for consumer information and finding a certified cognitive therapist

www.apahelpcenter.org
American Psychological Association website with articles and
  information for consumers

www.bazelon.org
Bazelon Center for Mental Health Law website with information
  pertaining to their work in national legal advocacy for the mentally ill

www.depressioncenter.net
An interactive website with online support available

www.dr-bob.org
Psychopharmacology tips

www.healthfinder.gov
U.S. Department of Health and Human Service sponsored site that connects to resources on the web pertaining to health related information.

www.human-nature.com
Clearing house for all aspects of human behavior

www.mentalhealth.org
U.S. Department of Health and Human Service website for mental health information

www.nacbt.org
National Association of Cognitive-Behavioral Therapists website with information for consumers and link to find a certified cognitive-behavioral therapist

www.naswdc.org/resources
National Association of Social Workers website with listing of social workers meeting national standards

www.psych.org/public_info/
American Psychiatric Association website with section on public information for patients

www.webmd.org
Website providing medical and health and wellness information

Appendix B

Medications Used in the Treatment of Bipolar Disorder

Medication generic (trade name)	Typical dosing range[1]	Max dosage recommended[2]	Available form	Cost/month[3]
Atypical antipsychotics				
Zyprexa, Zydis (olanzapine)	10–20 mg	20 mg	tab, liquid, injection	$360–$750
Risperdal (risperidone)	2–4 mg	6 mg	tab, liquid, injection	$140–$460
Seroquel (quetiapine)	200–800 mg	800 mg	tab	$200–$640
Geodon (ziprasidone)	80–160 mg	160 mg	cap, injection	$330–$360
Abilify (aripiprazole)	15–30 mg	30 mg	tab, liquid	$385–$545
Clozaril (clozapine)*	200–600 mg	900 mg	tab	$200–$600
Anticonvulsants				
Depakote, Depakote ER (valproate)	750–2000 mg (or 25mg/kg–60 mg/kg)	4000 mg	tab, cap, liquid	$120–$350
Tegretol*, Equetro (carbamazepine)	400–800 mg	1600 mg	tab, cap	$30–$200
Trileptal (oxcarbamazepine)*	1200–2400 mg	2400 mg	tab	$200–$450
Lamictil (lamotrigine)	200–400 mg	400 mg	tab	$155–$310
Topamax (topiramate)*	200–400 mg	1600 mg	tab	$200–$400
Neurontin (gabapentin)*	900–1800 mg	3600 mg	tab, cap, liquid	$130–$260
Gabitril (tiagabine)*	4–64 mg	64 mg	tab	$60–$500
Others				
Lithobid, Eskalith (lithium)	600–1200 mg	2400 mg	tab, cap	$15–$50
Symbyax (olanzapine/fluoxetine)	6/25–12/50 mg	18/75 mg	cap	$300–$440
Haldol (haloperidol)*	6–20 mg	100 mg	tab, liquid, injection	$40–$72
Trilafon (perphenazine)*	12–32 mg	64 mg	tab, liquid	$60–$95

*Does not have an FDA indication for bipolar disorder

[1]Average range for effective dose, but starting dose may be lower. Also, target doses may be reduced in children and older persons.

[2]Maximum dosage recommended is the manufacturer guideline that is FDA approved. In clinical practice, dosing may be higher.

[3]Costs are approximate only and based on generics if available with a range approximated from the cost of a 30-day supply of various doses within the typical dosing range listed for bipolar disorder per day. Although pills of various strengths are typically similar in cost, the need for half doses or two or more pills will result in greater cost, for example.

Appendix C

*Antidepressants**

*Antidepressants have an FDA indication for major depressive disorder, not bipolar depression.

Medication generic (trade name)	Typical dosing range[1]	Max Dosage Recommended[2]	Available Form	Cost/month[3]
SSRIs				
fluoxetine (Prozac)	20–60 mg	80 mg	tab, cap, liquid	$80–$250
sertraline (Zoloft)	50–200 mg	200 mg	tab, liquid	$80–$200
paroxetine (Paxil, CR)	20–75 mg	60 or 75 (CR) mg	tab, liquid	$100–$200
fluvoxamine (Luvox)	100–300 mg	300 mg	tab	$80–$240
citalopram (Celexa)	20–60 mg	60 mg	tab, liquid	$80–$160
escitalopram (Lexapro)	10–20 mg	20 mg	tab, liquid	$70–$110
TCAs				
clomipramine (Anfranil)	100–250 mg	250 mg	cap	$60–$150
amitriptyline (Elavil)	150–300 mg	300 mg	tab	$35–$100
doxepin (Sinequan)	150–300 mg	300 mg	cap, liquid	$35–$80
trimipramine (Surmontil)	150–300 mg	300 mg	cap	$80–$280
amoxepine	200–400 mg	600 mg	tab	$100–$200
protriptyline (Vivactil)	15–60 mg	60 mg	tab	$70–$280
desipramine (Norpramin)	150–300 mg	300 mg	tab	$65–$135
nortriptyline (Pamelor)	75–150 mg	150 mg	cap, liquid	$65–$130
imipramine (Tofranil)	150–300 mg	300 mg	tab	$60–$120
maprotiline (Ludiomil)	75–225 mg	225 mg	tab	$30–$85
MAOIs				
phenelzine (Nardil)	45–90 mg	90 mg	tab	$50–$100
tranylcypromine (Parnate)	30–60 mg	60 mg	tab	$75–$150

(continued)

Medication generic (trade name)	Typical dosing range[1]	Max Dosage Recommended[2]	Available Form	Cost/month[3]
Others				
trazodone (Desyrel)	150–600 mg	600 mg	tab	$45–$180
venlafaxine (Effexor, XR)	75–375 mg	375 or 225 (XR) mg	tab, cap	$60–$260
mirtazapine (Remeron)	15–45 mg	45 mg	tab	$80–$125
nefazodone (Serzone)	300–600 mg	600 mg	tab	$75–$150
bupropion (Wellbutrin, SR, XL)	300–450 mg	450 or 400 (SR) mg	tab	$85–$220
duloxetine (Cymbalta)	20–60 mg	60 mg	cap	$95–$200

[1]Average range for effective dose, but starting dose may be lower. Also, target doses may be reduced in children and older persons.

[2]Maximum dosage recommended is the manufacturer guideline that is FDA approved. In clinical practice, dosing may be higher.

[3]Costs are approximate only and based on generics if available with a range approximated from the cost of a 30-day supply of various doses within the typical dosing range listed for depression per day. While pills of various strengths are typically similar in cost, the need for half doses or 2 or more pills will result in greater cost, for example.

Appendix C

229

Glossary

Addiction: continued use of a mood-altering substance despite physical, psychological, or social harm. It is characterized by lack of control of amount and frequency of use, cravings, continued use in the presence of adverse effects, denial of negative consequences, and tendency to abuse other mood-altering substances.

Adoption study: a scientific study designed to control for genetic relatedness and environmental influences by comparing siblings adopted apart.

Affect: feeling or emotion, especially as manifested by facial expression or body language.

Affective flattening: a dulling of one's facial and emotional response to external stimuli.

Akathisia: a subjective sense of inner restlessness resulting in the need to keep moving. Objectively, restless movements or pacing may be signs of akathisia.

Algorithm: a sequence of steps to follow when approaching a particular problem.

Alogia: the inability to speak due to mental incapacity.

Alternative treatment: a treatment for a medical condition that has not undergone scientific studies to demonstrate its efficacy.

Anticonvulsant: a drug that controls or prevents seizures. Anticonvulsants are used in psychiatric practice to treat mania, mood instability, or other mental conditions.

Antidepressant: a drug specifically marketed for and capable of relieving the symptoms of clinical depression. Often used to treat conditions other than depression.

Antipsychotic: a drug that treats psychotic symptoms, such as hallucinations, delusions, and thought disorders. Antipsychotics can be used to treat certain mood disorders as well.

Anxiolytic: a substance that relieves subjective and objective symptoms of anxiety.

Attachment: the psychological connection between a child and his or her caretaker. Infants develop attachment behaviors within the first month. Deficits in early attachments can result in problems in later relationships in life.

Atypical antipsychotic: a second-generation antipsychotic with a profile of targeted brain receptors that differs from the older antipsychotics, which have fewer neurological side effects and also have mood-stabilizing effects.

Augmentation: in pharmacotherapy, a strategy of using a second medication to enhance the positive effects of an existing medication in the regimen.

Automatic thoughts: thoughts that occur spontaneously whenever a specific, common event occurs in one's life, and which are often associated with depression.

Autonomic nervous system: that part of the nervous system that is "involuntary" and is responsible for maintaining a relatively constant internal environment by controlling such involuntary functions as digestion, respiration, perspiration, and metabolism, as well as modulating blood pressure.

Avolition: a psychological state characterized by a general lack of desire, motivation, and persistence.

Axon: a single fiber of a nerve cell through which a message is sent via an electrical impulse to a receiving neuron. Each nerve cell has one axon.

Basal ganglia: a region of the brain consisting of three groups of nerve cells (called the caudate nucleus, putamen, and the globus pallidus) that are collectively responsible for control of movement. Abnormalities in the basal ganglia can result in involuntary movement disorders.

Benzodiazepine: a drug that is part of a class of medication with sedative and anxiolytic effects. Drugs in this class share a common chemical structure and mechanism of action.

Biogenic amines: a group of compounds in the nervous system that participate in the regulation of brain activity, which includes dopamine, serotonin, and norepinephrine.

Biopsychosocial: a model used to describe the possible origins of risk factors for the development of various mental illnesses, incorporating the biological, psychological, and societal factors for a given individual.

Bipolar depression: an episode of depression that occurs in the course of bipolar disorder.

Bipolar disorder: a mental illness defined by episodes of mania or hypomania, classically alternating with episodes of depression. There are, however, various forms the condition can take, such as repeated episodes of mania only, or lack of alternating episodes.

Catecholamines: a class of neurotransmitters in the brain that include epinephrine, norepineph-rine, and dopamine.

Cardiac toxicity: damage that occurs to the heart or coronary arteries as a result of medication side effects.

Catalepsy: A condition that occurs in a variety of physical and psychological disorders and is characterized by lack of response to external stimuli and by muscular rigidity, so that the limbs remain in whatever position they are placed.

Catastrophic thinking: a type of automatic thought during which the individual quickly assumes the worst outcome for a given situation.

Central nervous system: nerve cells and their support cells in the brain and spinal cord.

Chemical imbalance: a common vernacular for what is thought to be occurring in the brain in patients suffering from mental illness.

Cognitive-behavioral therapy: a combination of cognitive and behavioral approaches in psychotherapy, during which the therapist focuses on automatic thoughts and behavior of a self-defeating quality in order to make one more conscious of them and replace them with more positive thoughts and behaviors.

Comorbidity: the presence of two or more mental disorders, such as depression and anxiety.

Compliance: extent that behavior follows medical advice, such as by

taking prescribed treatments. Compliance can refer to medications as well as to appointments and psychotherapy sessions.

Concordance: in genetics, similarity in a twin pair with respect to presence or absence of illness.

Constitution: referring to a person's biopsychological make-up—that is, personality and traits.

Contingency contracting: a behavioral therapy technique that utilizes reinforcers or rewards to modify behaviors.

Countertransference: the attitudes, opinions, and behaviors that a therapist attributes to his or her patient, based not on the true nature of the patient but rather on the biased nature of the therapist because the patient reminds the therapist of his or her own past.

Defense mechanisms: a set of unconscious methods to protect one's personality from unpleasant thoughts and realities that may cause anxiety.

Delirium: a temporary state of mental confusion resulting from high fever, intoxication, shock, or other causes, and characterized by anxiety, disorientation, memory impairment, hallucinations, trembling, and incoherent speech.

Dependence: the body's reliance on a drug to function normally. Physical dependence results in withdrawal when the drug is stopped suddenly. Dependence should be contrasted with addiction.

Depression: a medical condition associated with changes in thoughts, moods, and behaviors.

Discontinuation syndrome: physical symptoms that occur when a drug is suddenly stopped.

Down-regulation: the reduction of receptors in a region of the brain in response to increased neurotransmitter in order to maintain homeostasis.

Dynamic: referring to a type of therapy that focuses on one's interpersonal relationships, developmental experiences, and the transference relationship with his or her therapist. Also known as insight-oriented.

Dysphoria: an emotional state of feeling unhappy or unwell.

Dyskinesia: an impairment in the ability to control movements.

Dysthymic: the presence of chronic, mild depressive symptoms.

ECT: Electroconvulsive or shock therapy.

Efficacy: the ability to produce a desired effect, such as the performance of a drug or therapy in relieving symptoms.

Ego-dystonic: that which is unacceptable to the self (ego).

Ego-syntonic: that which is acceptable to the self (ego).

Electrochemically: the way in which signals are transmitted neurologically. Brain chemicals, or neurotransmitters, alter the electrical conductivity of nerve tissue, causing a signal to be transmitted.

Endocrine disorder: a disorder of the endocrine system. Endocrine glands release chemicals (also known as hormones), whose actions occur at another site, directly into the blood stream. Endocrine glands include the thyroid, ovaries and testes, adrenals, and pancreas.

Endocrine glands: ductless glands in the body that synthesize and secrete chemical messengers (hormones) into the blood stream or lymph for transport to target cells.

Enzyme: a protein made in the body that serves to break down or create other molecules. Enzymes serve as catalysts to biochemical reactions in the body.

Extrapyramidal: the parts of the brain responsible for static motor control. The basal ganglia are part of this system. Deficits in this system result in involuntary movement disorders. Antipsychotic medications affect these areas, leading to extrapyramidal side effects, which include muscle spasms (dystonias), tremors, shuffling gait, restlessness (akathisia), and tardive dyskinesias.

Fight or flight: a reaction in the body that occurs in response to an immediate threat. Adrenaline is released, which allows for rapid energy to run (flight) or to face the threat (fight).

First-degree relative: immediate biologically related family member, such as biological parents or full siblings.

Flight of ideas: a type of thought disorder in which there is repeated switch of topic either mid-sentence or inappropriate to the topic at hand.

Flooding: a behavioral therapy technique that involves exposure to the maximal level of anxiety as quickly as possible.

Free association: the mental process of saying out loud whatever comes to mind, suppressing the natural tendency to censor or filter thoughts. This technique is utilized in psychoanalysis and in psychodynamic psychotherapy.

Functional: generally referring to a symptom or condition that has no clearly defined physiological or anatomical cause.

Gene: DNA sequence that codes for a specific protein or that regulates other genes. Genes are heritable.

Graded exposure: a psychotherapeutic technique applied to rid a patient of specific phobias. A gradual exposure to the phobic situation is set about first through imagery techniques, then through limited exposure in time and intensity before full exposure occurs.

Grandiosity: the tendency to consider the self or one's ideas better or more superior to what is reality.

Gray matter: the part of the brain that contains the nerve cell bodies, including the cell nucleus and its metabolic machinery, as opposed to the axons, which are essentially the "transmission wires" of the nerve cell. The cerebral cortex contains gray matter.

Half-life: the time it takes for half of the blood concentration of a medication to be eliminated from the body. Half-life determines as well the time

to equilibrium of a drug in the blood and determines the frequency of dosing to achieve that equilibrium.

Hepatitis: inflammation of the liver, caused by infection or toxin.

Homeostasis: the maintenance of relatively stable internal physiological conditions in the body.

Hormonal: referring to the chemicals that are secreted by the endocrine glands and act throughout the body.

Hyperarousal: a heightened state of alertness to external and internal stimuli, often resulting in sleep disturbance, problems concentrating, hypervigilance, and exaggerated startle response. Typically seen in post-traumatic conditions.

Hypersomnia: an inability to stay awake. Oversleeping.

Hypomanic: milder form of mania with the same symptoms but of lesser intensity.

Hypopnea: abnormally slow, shallow breathing.

Hypothyroidism: decreased or absence of thyroid hormone, which is secreted by an endocrine gland near the throat and has wide metabolic effects. When thyroid hormone is low, metabolism can slow, leading to symptoms that can mimic clinical depression.

Indoleamines: a class of neurotransmitters in the brain that includes serotonin.

Insight-oriented: see *dynamic*. A form of psychotherapy that focuses on one's developmental history, interpersonal relationships with one's family of origin, and current relationships with friends, spouses, and others. Usually such relationships are explored through the development of a transference relationship with one's therapist.

Informed consent: the premise that patients have a right to determine what happens to their body, and as such agreement to a treatment requires receipt of information, competence to make the decision, and agreeability for the treatment.

Interpersonal therapy: a form of therapy. Unlike insight-oriented or dynamic therapy that focuses on developmental relationships, interpersonal therapy focuses strictly on current relationships and conflicts within them.

Interpersonal social rhythm therapy: a form of therapy based on the principles of interpersonal therapy. Specifically geared toward the treatment of bipolar disorder with monitoring of daily activities, including sleep.

Insomnia: the inability to fall asleep, middle-of-the-night awakening, or early morning awakening.

Kindling: changes that occur in the brain as a result of repeated intermittent exposure to a subthreshold electrical or chemical stimulus (such as in seizures) so that there develops a permanent decrease in the threshold of excitability.

Leucopenia: an abnormal lowering of the white blood cell count.

Limbic system: the part of the brain thought to be related to feeding, mating, and most importantly to emotion and memory of emotional events. Brain regions within this system include the hypothalamus, hippocampus, amygdala, and cingulate gyrus as well as portions of the basal ganglia.

Malignant hypertension: elevated blood pressure that is acute and rapidly progressive with severe symptoms, including headache.

Mania: a condition characterized by elevation of mood (extreme euphoria or irritability) associated with racing thoughts, decreased need for sleep, hyperactivity, and poor impulse control. One episode of mania (in the absence of an ingested substance) is needed to diagnose bipolar disorder.

Mental illness: a medical condition defined by functional symptoms with as yet no specific pathophysiology that impairs social, academic, and occupational function.

Mental status: snapshot portrait of one's cognitive and emotional functioning at a particular point in time. It is always included as part of a psychiatric examination.

Metabolize: the process of breaking down a drug in the blood.

Mood disorder: a type of mental illness that affects mood primarily and cognition secondarily. Mood disorders predominantly consist of depression and bipolar disorder.

Mood-incongruent: symptoms that are inconsistent with the dominant mood state, such as euphoria in the presence of paranoia of being harmed.

Mood stabilizer: typically refers to medications for the treatment and prevention of mood swings, such as from depression to mania.

Morbidity: the impact a particular disease process or illness has on one's social, academic, or occupational functioning.

Mortality: death secondary to illness or disease.

Motor cortex: portion of the cerebral cortex that is directly related to voluntary movement. Also known as the motor strip, its anatomy correlates accurately with specific bodily movements, such as moving the left upper or lower extremities.

Neuroanatomy: the structural make-up of the nervous system and nervous tissue.

Neurological: referring to all matters of the nervous system that includes brain, brain stem, spinal cord and peripheral nerves. Problems with specific, identifiable pathophysiological processes are generally considered to be neurological as opposed to psychiatric. Problems with elements of both pathophysiological and psychiatric manifestations are considered to be neuro-psychiatric.

Neuron: a nerve cell made up of a cell body with extensions called the dendrites and the axon. The dendrites carry messages from the synapse to the cell body, and the axon carries messages to the synapse to communicate with other nerve cells.

Neuronal plasticity: the act of nerve growth and change as a result of learning. Mental exercise alters neuronal growth in the same manner physical exercise alters muscle growth.

Neurophysiology: the part of science devoted specifically to the physiology, or function and activities, of the nervous system.

Neurotransmitter: chemical in the brain that is released by nerve cells to send a message to other cells via the cell receptors.

Norepinephrine: a neurotransmitter that is involved in the regulation of mood, arousal, and memory.

Numbing: the psychological process of becoming resistant to external stimuli so that previously pleasurable activities become less desirable.

Off-label: prescribing of a medication for indications other than those outlined by the Food and Drug Administration (FDA).

Overgeneralization: the act of taking a specific event, usually psychologically traumatic, and applying one's reactions to that event to an ever-increasing array of events that are not really in the same class but are perceived as such.

Pancreatitis: inflammation of the pancreas.

Parasympathetic nervous system: that part of the autonomic nervous system that allows for rest, recovery, and storage of new energy in the body between stressful situations.

Paresthesias: presence of numbness and tingling in limbs. Often a symptom in anxiety disorders.

Personality disorder: maladaptive behavior patterns that persist throughout the life span that cause functional impairments.

Pharmacological: pertaining to all chemicals that, when ingested, cause a physiological process to occur in the body. Psychopharmacological refers to those physiological processes that have direct psychological effects.

Physiological: pertaining to functions and activities of the living matter, such as organs, tissues, or cells.

Placebo: an inert substance that when ingested causes absolutely no physiological process to occur but may have psychological effects.

Postpartum: referring to events occurring within a specified time after giving birth. Usually within the first four weeks.

Pressured speech: characterized by the need to keep speaking; it is difficult to interrupt someone with this type of speech. Commonly seen in manic or hypomanic mood states.

Prevalence: ratio of the frequency of cases in the population in a given time period of a particular event to the number of persons in the population at risk for the event.

Projected: the attribution of one's own unconscious thoughts and feelings to others.

Prophylaxis: the prevention of disease.

Psychomotor agitation: hyperactive or restless movement. Can be seen in highly anxious states, manic mood states, or intoxicated states.

Psychomotor retarded: slowed movement, usually as a result of severe clinical depression. When emotion and cognition become depressed enough, motor function can also become depressed, causing such a phenomenon.

Psychosocial: pertaining to environmental circumstances that can impact one's psychological well-being.

Psychotropic: usually referring to pharmacological agents (medications) that, as a result of their physiological effects on the brain, lead to direct psychological effects.

Racing thoughts: the subjective feeling of having thoughts in one's mind move quickly from one topic to the next, often difficult to follow and make sense of, typically associated with rapid, uninterruptible speech.

Rational polypharmacy: the practice of combination medication therapy with consideration of the clinical effects, adverse effects, drug interactions, and relation between effective and toxic drug levels, as well as with an understanding of the mechanisms of action of each agent.

Receptor: a protein on a cell upon which specific chemicals from within the body or from the environment bind, in order to cause changes in the cell that result in an electrochemical message for a certain action to be taken by that cell.

Recovery: achievement of baseline, premorbid functioning after successful treatment for a mental illness. *Recovery* is the term used after a time period of six months symptom free. Up to that point the term used is *remission*.

Recurrence: the return of symptoms of a mental illness following complete recovery, considered to have occurred following a period of six months symptom free.

Re-experiencing: the phenomenon of having a previous lived experience vividly recalled and accompanied by the same strong emotions one originally experienced.

Refractory depression: depressive illness that does not respond to a therapeutic intervention. The term is not typically applied unless such a lack of response has occurred to several different interventions.

Relapse: the return of symptoms of a mental illness for which one is currently receiving active treatment. Relapse occurs during response to treatment or during remission of symptoms. If symptoms recur after six months of successful treatment during what is termed the recovery phase, the term used is *recurrence*.

Relative risk: a ratio of incidence of a disorder in persons exposed to a risk factor to the incidence of a disorder in persons not exposed to the same risk factor.

Remission: complete cessation of all symptoms associated with a specific

mental illness. This occurs within the first six months of treatment, after which the term used is *recovery*.

Resistance: the tendency to avoid treatment interventions, often unconsciously (e.g., missing appointments, arriving late, forgetting medication).

Response: referring to at least a 50% reduction but not complete cessation of all symptoms associated with a specific mental illness, such as depression.

Ruminations: obsessive thinking over an idea or decision.

Schema: representations in the mind of the world that affect perception of and response to the environment.

Second-generation antipsychotic: see *atypical antipsychotic.*

Serotonin: a neurotransmitter found in the brain and throughout the body. Serotonin is involved in mood regulation, anxiety, pain perception, appetite, sleep, sexual behavior, and impulsive behavior.

Serotonin syndrome: an extremely rare but life-threatening syndrome associated with the direct physiological effects of serotonin overload on the body. Symptoms include flushing, high fever, tachycardia, and seizures.

Somatic: referring to the body. Somatic therapy refers to all treatments that have direct physiological effects, such as medication and ECT. Somatic complaints refer to all physical complaints that refer to the body, such as aches and pains.

Somnambulism: sleepwalking.

Splitting: a defense mechanism that serves to separate opposing affective or emotional states, such as in overidealizing a person one day and devaluing the same person the next. The ability for the ego to hold more than one representation of an object is impaired. Splitting can describe the process of dividing the members of a treatment team in regards to the work with a mutual patient.

Stevens-Johnson syndrome: a severe inflammatory eruption of the skin and mucous membranes that can occur as an allergic reaction to a medication.

Stressors: environmental influences on the body and mind that can have gradual adverse effects.

Subsyndromal: exhibiting symptoms that are not severe enough to be characterized as a syndrome.

Sympathetic nervous system: the part of the autonomic nervous system that is responsible for providing responses and energy needed to cope with stressful situations such as fear or extremes of physical activity.

Synaptic cleft: the junction between two neurons where neurotransmitters are released thereby continuing or changing communication.

Tarasoff: the name of a family that sued the therapist involved in the care of a young man who murdered a family member. As a result of the lawsuit, therapists are now required to protect and warn potential victims from violent acts or threats made by patients under their care.

Tardive dyskinesia: a late-onset involuntary movement disorder, often irreversible, typically of the mouth, tongue, or lips, and less commonly of the limbs and trunk. These movements are a consequence of antipsychotic use but are less commonly observed with the newer, atypical antipsychotics.

Teratogenic: that which can interfere with normal embryonic development.

Therapeutic index: the ratio between the toxic dose and the therapeutic dose of a drug, used as a measure of the relative safety of the drug for a particular treatment.

Thought stopping: a technique used to suppress repetitive thoughts.

Thrombocytopenia: an abnormal decrease in the number of platelets in the blood.

Transference: the unconscious assignment of feelings and attitudes to a therapist from previous important relationships in one's life (parents and siblings). The relationship follows the pattern of its prototype and can be either negative or positive. The transference relationship is a critical event for the progress of a patient in insight-oriented, or psychodynamic, therapy.

Treatment plan: the plan agreed upon by patient and clinician that will be implemented to treat a mental illness. It incorporates all modalities (therapy and medication).

Unconscious: an underlying motivation for behavior that is not available to the conscious or thoughtful mind, which has developed over the course of life experience.

Unipolar: in contrast to manic-depressive illness, known as *bi*polar, or two poles of mood states, the description of major depression, or the presence of one pole of mood state.

Up-regulation: the increase of receptors in a region of the brain in response to a reduction of neurotransmitter in order to maintain homeostasis.

Visceral: a bodily sensation usually referencing the gut. Also a feeling or thought attributed to intuition rather than reason, such as a "gut instinct."

White matter: tracts in the brain that consist of sheaths (called myelin) covering long nerve fibers.

Index

Index